NATIONAL ACADEMIES *Sciences* *Engineering* *Medicine*

NATIONAL
ACADEMIES
PRESS
Washington, DC

Health Disparities in the Medical Record and Disability Determinations

T0357694

Austen Applegate, Carol Mason Spicer,
and Joe Alper, *Rapporteurs*

Board on Health Care Services

Health and Medicine Division

Proceedings of a Workshop

NATIONAL ACADEMIES PRESS 500 Fifth Street, NW Washington, DC 20001

This activity was supported by a contract (28321323D00060012) between the National Academy of Sciences and the Social Security Administration. Any opinions, findings, conclusions, or recommendations expressed in this publication do not necessarily reflect the views of any organization or agency that provided support for the project.

International Standard Book Number-13: 978-0-309-72444-9
International Standard Book Number-10: 0-309-72444-9
Digital Object Identifier: https://doi.org/10.17226/27909

This publication is available from the National Academies Press, 500 Fifth Street, NW, Keck 360, Washington, DC 20001; (800) 624-6242 or (202) 334-3313; http://www.nap.edu.

Suggested citation: National Academies of Sciences, Engineering, and Medicine. 2024. *Health disparities in the medical record and disability determinations: Proceedings of a workshop.* Washington, DC: The National Academies Press. https://doi.org/10.17226/27909.

The **National Academy of Sciences** was established in 1863 by an Act of Congress, signed by President Lincoln, as a private, nongovernmental institution to advise the nation on issues related to science and technology. Members are elected by their peers for outstanding contributions to research. Dr. Marcia McNutt is president.

The **National Academy of Engineering** was established in 1964 under the charter of the National Academy of Sciences to bring the practices of engineering to advising the nation. Members are elected by their peers for extraordinary contributions to engineering. Dr. John L. Anderson is president.

The **National Academy of Medicine** (formerly the Institute of Medicine) was established in 1970 under the charter of the National Academy of Sciences to advise the nation on medical and health issues. Members are elected by their peers for distinguished contributions to medicine and health. Dr. Victor J. Dzau is president.

The three Academies work together as the **National Academies of Sciences, Engineering, and Medicine** to provide independent, objective analysis and advice to the nation and conduct other activities to solve complex problems and inform public policy decisions. The National Academies also encourage education and research, recognize outstanding contributions to knowledge, and increase public understanding in matters of science, engineering, and medicine.

Learn more about the National Academies of Sciences, Engineering, and Medicine at **www.nationalacademies.org**.

PLANNING COMMITTEE FOR THE WORKSHOP ON HEALTH DISPARITIES IN THE MEDICAL RECORD AND DISABILITY DETERMINATIONS[1]

AMY J. HOUTROW (*Cochair*), Professor and Vice Chair, University of Pittsburgh School of Medicine

KARRIE A. SHOGREN (*Cochair*), Ross and Marianna Beach Distinguished Professor, University of Kansas

KENRICK CATO, Professor of Informatics, Children's Hospital of Philadelphia

KENSAKU KAWAMOTO, Professor of Biomedical Informatics, University of Utah

ELHAM MAHMOUDI, Associate Professor of Health Economics, University of Michigan

JONATHAN PLATT, Assistant Professor of Epidemiology, University of Iowa

AMANDA ALISE PRICE, Director, Office of Health Equity, and Chief Scientific Diversity Officer, Eunice Kennedy Shriver National Institute of Child Health and Human Development

MICHAEL V. STANTON, Associate Professor, California State University, East Bay

RUPA VALDEZ, Professor, University of Virgina

RUQAIIJAH YEARBY, Kara J. Trott Professor in Health Law at Moritz College of Law, The Ohio State University

Staff

CAROL MASON SPICER, Senior Program Officer
AUSTEN APPLEGATE, Research Associate
CHIDINMA CHUKWURAH, Senior Program Assistant
JULIE WILTSHIRE, Senior Finance Business Partner

---

[1] The planning committee's role was limited to planning the workshop, and the Proceedings of a Workshop has been prepared by the workshop rapporteurs with assistance from the National Academies staff as a factual summary of what occurred at the workshop. Statements, recommendations, and opinions expressed are those of individual presenters and participants and are not necessarily endorsed or verified by the National Academies of Sciences, Engineering, and Medicine, and they should not be construed as reflecting any group consensus.

ELISE MIALOU, Senior Finance Business Partner
SHARYL NASS, Senior Board Director

Consultant

JOE ALPER, Science Writer

LINDA D. SCOTT, Dean and Professor, University of Wisconsin-Madison School of Nursing

HARDEEP SINGH, Chief, Health Policy Quality and Informatics Program, Center for Innovations in Quality Effectiveness and Safety, Michael E. DeBakey VA Medical Center

HEMI TEWARSON, Executive Director, National Academy for State and Health Policy

KEEGAN D. WARREN, Executive Director, Institute for Healthcare Access, Texas A&M University

LAURIE ZEPHYRIN, Senior Vice President, Advancing Health Equity, The Commonwealth Fund

MICHAEL ZUBKOFF, Director, MD-MBA Program, Dartmouth; Associate Dean, Geisel School of Medicine, and Faculty Director, Center for Health Care, Tuck School of Business at Dartmouth

Reviewers

This Proceedings of a Workshop was reviewed in draft form by individuals chosen for their diverse perspectives and technical expertise. The purpose of this independent review is to provide candid and critical comments that will assist the National Academies of Sciences, Engineering, and Medicine in making each published proceedings as sound as possible and to ensure that it meets the institutional standards for quality, objectivity, evidence, and responsiveness to the charge. The review comments and draft manuscript remain confidential to protect the integrity of the process.

We thank the following individuals for their review of this proceedings:

KATHLEEN L. KANE, Kane Law, LLC
KENSAKU KAWAMOTO, University of Utah
TARA LAGU, Northwestern University Feinberg School of Medicine

Although the reviewers listed above provided many constructive comments and suggestions, they were not asked to endorse the content of the proceedings nor did they see the final draft before its release. The review of this proceedings was overseen by **PAUL VOLBERDING,** University of California San Francisco. He was responsible for making certain that an independent examination of this proceedings was carried out in accordance with standards of the National Academies and that all review comments were carefully considered. Responsibility for the final content rests entirely with the rapporteurs and the National Academies.

We also thank staff member **LIDA BENINSON** for reading and providing helpful comments on this manuscript.

Acknowledgments

The National Academies of Sciences, Engineering, and Medicine's Standing Committee of Medical and Vocational Experts for the Social Security Administration's Disability Programs wishes to express its sincere gratitude to the planning committee cochairs Amy J. Houtrow and Karrie A. Shogren for their valuable contributions to the development and orchestration of this workshop. The standing committee wishes to thank all the members of the planning committee who collaborated to ensure a workshop complete with information presentations and rich discussions. The standing committee also wishes to thank the speakers, who generously shared their time and expertise with workshop participants. Finally, this project was funded with generous support from the Social Security Administration, which is critical to the success of the Standing Committee of Medical and Vocational Experts for the Social Security Administration's Disability Programs.

Contents

Boxes and Figures

Acronyms and Abbreviations

ADA   Americans with Disabilities Act of 1990
AI   artificial intelligence

BRIDGE   Broadening the Reach, Impact, and Delivery of Genetic Services trial

CDC   Centers for Disease Control and Prevention

DDS   Disability Determination Services

EHR   electronic health record

FQHC   federally qualified health center

HHS   Department of Health and Human Services

ICD   International Classification of Diseases
IT   information technology

NIH   National Institutes of Health
NLP   natural language processing

SDOH   social determinants of health
SGA   substantial gainful activity

SSA	Social Security Administration
SSDI	Social Security Disability Insurance
SSI	Supplemental Security Income

1

Introduction

The Social Security Administration (SSA) administers two programs that provide cash payments to people with disabilities: the Social Security Disability Insurance (SSDI) program and the Supplemental Security Income (SSI) program. Disability insurance aims to protect workers contributing to the program through payroll tax deductions from lost earnings arising because of impairment, while SSI's goal is to guarantee a base income for the poorest of the aged, blind, or disabled population (Meseguer, 2013). SSA relies on a network of local SSA field offices and state-run, federally funded agencies called Disability Determination Services (DDSs) to process disability claims. After the field offices verify nonmedical eligibility requirements, the DDSs develop the medical evidence to support a disability claim using evidence from the individual's electronic health record (EHR).

Medical records are not perfect, however, particularly in the manner in which they represent disparities in access to care, the availability of specialists, and social determinants of health. They can also be flawed because of clinician bias, whether explicit or implicit, as reflected in the language they use when describing an individual's condition. These inequities and disparities can hinder SSA disability determinations.

To better understand the effect of health inequities and the manner in which they affect SSA's disability programs, the Health and Medicine Division of the National Academies of Sciences, Engineering, and Medicine hosted a 1.5-day workshop on April 4–5, 2024, that examined the variety of different experiences with the U.S. health care system common to individuals with disabilities facing barriers—including members of racial or ethnic minorities, people with low income, people who have limited English proficiency, those facing homelessness, or people with mental illness—and the consequences of those different experiences on an individual's health status, medical record, and SSA disability determinations. Box 1-1 provides the statement of task for the workshop, which SSA funded.

BOX 1-1
Statement of Task

A planning committee of the National Academies of Sciences, Engineering, and Medicine will plan and host a public workshop on the variety of different experiences with the U.S. healthcare system common to individuals facing barriers,[a] including members of racial or ethnic minorities, and the consequences of those different experiences on an individual's health status and medical record, which is relevant to the U.S. Social Security Administration (SSA) in disability determinations. The workshop shall include presentations with a focus on how individual's different experiences can manifest in records, as well as medical advances, developments, and research related to health inequities in the United States.

The workshop will feature invited presentations and panel discussions on topics such as:

- The primary social determinants of health affecting people facing barriers and members of racial or ethnic minorities, how they might be reflected in medical records, and how they differ between and among various groups.
- Societal, systemic, racial, cultural, or personal characteristics that can serve as impediments to people facing barriers and members of racial or ethnic minorities seeking or receiving medical services and, in particular:
  a. How those characteristics may be recorded or manifest in traditional and other healthcare records;
  b. How the medical records of people with those characteristics might differ from the general population; and
  c. How the impact of those impediments can be lessened or averted, particularly in the context of consultative examinations ordered by SSA.
- The lived experiences of people facing barriers and members of racial or ethnic minorities as they interact with SSA,

---

BOX 1-1 Continued

healthcare systems, and alternative sources of medical care, including:

a. How those experiences impact future use of or trust in medical or healthcare services;

b. Disconnects between the health-related reports made by people facing barriers and the information recorded by their healthcare providers;

c. Are there alternative sources of medical care utilized by some people facing barriers; and

d. Areas of difficulty or confusion when making a disability application, providing SSA with medical and other records, or attending a consultative examination.

- An overview of recent or emerging research suggesting particular widely-used tests or procedures are not as accurate or appropriate as traditionally believed for certain sub-populations and, for each, whether alternate tests or procedures exist which have been found to be accurate and appropriate for the population in question.

The planning committee shall develop the agenda for the workshop sessions, select and invite speakers and discussants, and moderate the discussions. The speakers and discussants will have the experience and knowledge to speak to the differences experienced by various racial and ethnic populations and other groups of people facing barriers. A proceedings of the presentations and discussions at the workshop will be prepared by a designated rapporteur in accordance with institutional guidelines.

---

[a] Including people with low income, limited English proficiency, facing homelessness, or with mental illness.

As Michael Goldstein, director of SSA's Office of Disability Policy, noted in his introductory remarks to the workshop, inequities in providing health care services are "an unfortunate reality" of the U.S. health care system. He explained that understanding the effect of health disparities on SSA's disability programs requires understanding where these disparities come from and how they affect the accuracy of an individual's medical record, saying

We need that information first, to be able to identify [affected] cases, and second, to unravel the accurate from the misleading evidence within those cases, which I am not disillusioned will be an easy process.

He added that SSA does provide guidance to health care providers on the types of evidence SSA needs to make a disability determination, and it offers questionnaires that claimants or people who know them well can complete. "Ultimately, our adjudicators consider all the evidence in an individual's case, not just medical evidence and not just that from doctors or other health care providers."

This Proceedings of a Workshop summarizes the presentations and discussions, reflecting the speakers', panelists', and participants' broad range of views and ideas. The speakers' presentations (as PDFs and video files) are available online.[1]

---

[1] The workshop speakers' presentations are available at https://www.nationalacademies.org/event/41744_04-2024_health-disparities-in-the-medical-record-and-disability-determinations-a-workshop.

2

Overview, Concepts, and Framing

Key Messages from Individual Speakers

- The medical model of disability locates the problem of disability at the person, and it operates in the context of disease, disorders, and impairments. The social model of disability understands disabilities in terms of attitudinal barriers, barriers in the built environment, and noninclusive practices that work together to prevent people with impairments from participating in various activities. (Houtrow)
- The Social Security Administration's (SSA's) disability programs are not driven by diagnoses but are evidence- or impairment-driven programs. (Nibali)
- Achieving health equity is not a finite project that will be implemented or completed in a predictable period of time. It requires a constant process and engaging a cycle of improvement that actively engages those most affected in all stages of the process. (Platt)
- Billing is at the core of electronic health records, but today they are central to clinical care, quality reporting, and regulatory compliance, serving as accessible repositories of patient information and supporting clinical decision making. Clinical decision support is an increasingly important function of electronic health records. (Kawamoto)

The workshop's first session provided a high-level overview of topics that served as background for the rest of the workshop. The four speakers in this session were Amy J. Houtrow, professor and vice chair in the Department of Physical Medicine and Rehabilitation for Pediatric Rehabilitation Medicine at the University of Pittsburgh School of Medicine; Vincent Nibali, policy analyst at the Social Security Administration (SSA); Jonathan Platt, assistant professor at the University of Iowa College of Public Health; and Kensaku Kawamoto, associate chief medical information officer at University of Utah Health and professor and vice chair of clinical informatics in the University of Utah's Department of Biomedical Informatics.

DEFINITION OF DISABILITY

Houtrow began her presentation by displaying a thought bubble containing words people might associate with disability, depending on their perspective (Figure 2-1). She explained:

> From a doctoring perspective, we might think of a health condition or a disorder or a disease. From a person's body and how it works, we might think of impairments. And people with disabilities often think of disability as identity.

In the academic world, the *International Classification of Functioning, Disability and Health* provides a useful framework for framing and understanding disability (Figure 2-2) and the experiences of people with disabilities

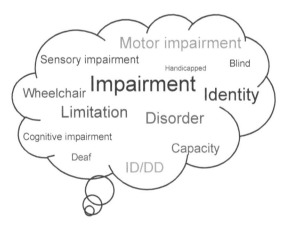

FIGURE 2-1 A thought bubble with words people might associate with disability.
SOURCE: Houtrow presentation, April 4, 2024.

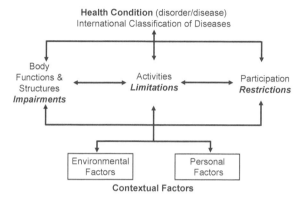

FIGURE 2-2 The *International Classification of Functioning, Disability and Health* model of disability.
SOURCES: Houtrow presentation, April 4, 2024; World Health Organization (WHO). 2001. CC BY-NC-SA 3.0 IGO.

(World Health Organization, 2001). Clinicians use the International Classification of Diseases (ICD) to classify the myriad diseases, disorders, and conditions that affect humans. Environmental and personal factors interact with an individual's health condition and contextualize people's experiences. Houtrow said:

> When we think about a health condition, we are thinking about impairments at the body level, activity limitations in what someone does, and participation restriction and how they are able to engage successfully as desired in society.

Houtrow explained the difference between the medical and social models of disability. The medical model locates the problem of disability at the person, and it operates in the context of disease, disorders, and impairments. The social model understands disabilities in terms of attitudinal barriers, barriers in the built environment and noninclusive practices that work together to prevent people with impairments from participating in various activities.

The Centers for Disease Control and Prevention (CDC) defines disability as

> Any condition of the body or mind (impairment) that makes it more difficult for the person with the condition to do certain activities (activity limitation) and interact with the world around them (participation restrictions). (CDC, 2024)

Based on this definition, CDC estimates that 27 percent of U.S. adults have a disability. According to the Americans with Disabilities Act of 1990 (ADA), a person with a disability is someone who has a physical or mental impairment that substantially limits one or more major life activities.[1] This includes people who have a history or record of such an impairment or a person others perceive as having such an impairment (Civil Rights Division, 2008).

Houtrow said meeting SSA's definition of disability requires an individual be unable to engage in any substantial gainful activity because of a medically determinable physical or mental impairment expected to lead to death or that has lasted or is expected to last for a continuous period of at least twelve months. Making that determination requires objective medical evidence and laboratory findings, among other considerations. SSA considers children to be disabled if the child has a medically determinable physical or mental impairment or combination of these two factors, if the impairment results in marked and severe functional limitations, and if the impairment has lasted, or is expected to last, for at least one year or until death. Domains of activity for assessing a child's functioning include acquiring and using information, attending to and completing tasks, interacting and relating with others, moving about and manipulating objects, caring for one's self, and health and physical well-being.

Houtrow commented on the language for discussing disability. Person-first language, such as "Amy is a person with disabilities," shifts the focus from the impairment to the social barriers that impede full participation in society as desired. Identity-first language, such as "I am a disabled woman," treats the disability as a cultural identity from which the individual cannot separate themself. Houtrow said:

> There are ongoing conversations about when and where this language should be used, and it is really about a shared common goal to recognize, affirm, and validate all of our identities in personhood and to recognize people with disabilities as equal members in our society. Today you will hear both, and both are deemed acceptable.

OVERVIEW OF SSA'S DISABILITY DETERMINATION PROCESS

Vincent Nibali explained that while the Social Security Disability Insurance (SSDI) and Supplemental Security Income (SSI) programs have different non-medical eligibility requirements, both have the same medical and vocational eligibility requirements and both are only for individuals with a complete disability

---

[1] Major life activities include eating, sleeping, speaking, breathing, walking, standing, lifting, bending, thinking and concentrating, seeing and hearing, and working, reading, learning, and communicating.

that leaves the individual unable to work. SSA defines disability for adults as the inability to engage in any substantial gainful activity (SGA) because of a medically determinable physical or mental impairment that will likely result in death or that has lasted or that will likely last for a continuous period of not less than twelve months. SGA is an SSA term defined by earnings per month. For 2024, the value for SGA is $1,550 or more per month and $2,590 for blind individuals.

To determine if an adult meets the requirement to be unable to engage in SGA, SSA has a five-step, sequential evaluation process that allows it to make a disability decision at the earliest possible step without prejudicing any claimants:

1. Is the individual engaged in SGA?
2. Is the impairment a medically determinable physical or mental impairment that is severe, and does it meet the duration requirement (see Box 2-1)?
3. Does the individual's medical condition meet or medically equal a listing, where listings are publicly available sets of criteria for specific impairments that SSA believes represent a higher level of limitation than the program requires in general (see Box 2-2)?
4. Does the impairment prevent the individual from performing their past relevant work?
5. Does the individual have the ability to adjust to other work?

BOX 2-1
Definition of Terms Relevant to
Determining Impairment Severity

- Medically determinable impairment: An impairment must result from anatomical, physiological, or psychological abnormalities that can be shown by medically acceptable clinical and laboratory diagnostic techniques. Therefore, a physical or mental impairment must be established by objective medical evidence from an acceptable medical source.
- Objective medical evidence: Signs, laboratory findings, or both.
- Acceptable medical source: A licensed physician or psychologist, or when within the scope of their practice, an optometrist, podiatrist, speech-language pathologist, audiologist, licensed advanced practice registered nurse, or licensed physician assistant.

SOURCE: Nibali presentation, April 4, 2024.

BOX 2-2
Listings of Impairments

Listings of impairments describe for each of the major body systems impairments that SSA considers to be severe enough to prevent an individual from doing any gainful activity, regardless of age, education, or work experience. In the case of children under age 18, the impairment must be severe enough to cause marked and severe functional limitations. The listings are special rules that provide SSA with a mechanism to identify claims that it should clearly allow. An impairment (or combination of impairments) is medically equal to a listed impairment in the listings if it is at least equal in severity and duration to the criteria of any listed impairment.

SOURCE: Nibali presentation, April 4, 2024.

Nibali explained that if an individual meets the criteria of a listing, SSA will find them disabled at Step 3, with no need to proceed to Steps 4 and 5. However, SSA will never find someone is not disabled if they do not meet the Step 3 criteria. He also noted that SSA's disability programs are not driven by diagnoses but are evidence- or impairment-driven programs. "Just because a doctor has never signed on the line diagnosing you with a specific condition does not mean we cannot consider that condition or the underlying limitations from it," said Nibali. Before moving to Steps 4 and 5, SSA determines an individual's "residual functional capacity," the most a claimant can do, despite their limitations. This determination is based on all relevant evidence in the case record and considers all medical determinable impairments, even those that are not severe.

To define the work requirements for Steps 4 and 5, SSA has used the 1991 edition of the *Dictionary of Occupational Titles*. However, because this publication has not been updated, SSA is working with the Bureau of Labor and Statistics to collect data and develop a new set of vocational requirements it will use for Steps 4 and 5.

For children, SSA uses a different set of criteria that includes:

- A medically determinable physical or mental impairment or combination of impairments that causes marked and severe functional limitations, and that will likely result in death or that has lasted or will likely last for a continuous period of not less than twelve months; and

- An impairment (or impairments) causes marked and severe functional limitations if it meets or medically equals the severity of a set of criteria for an impairment in the listings, or if it functionally equals the listings.

In the adjudication process for a child's disability, SSA follows the first two steps in the adult process, but for Step 3, SSA adds the concept of "functionally equals the listings."[2] Nibali specified the term *functionally equals the listing* means an impairment must be of listing-level severity that results in marked limitations in two domains of functioning or an extreme limitation in one domain compared to children of the same age without impairments. The six relevant domains are acquiring and using information, attending to and completing tasks, interacting and relating with others, moving about and manipulating objects, caring for oneself, and health and physical well-being.

BASICS OF HEALTH DISPARITIES

Jonathan Platt began his presentation by defining key terms and concepts relevant to health disparities and describing potential steps to achieve health equity (see Box 2-3 and Figure 2-3). He noted that people with disabilities experience a range of disparities. For example, while people with disabilities account for 11.7 percent of the school population, they account for 25 percent of all suspensions, 23 percent of all expulsions, and 27 percent of all arrests at school. Black students, who make up 19 percent of students with disabilities, account for 36 percent of suspended students with disabilities (Nowicki, 2018). In addition, people with disabilities are twice as likely to be unemployed (Office of Disability Employment Policy, 2024) and are more likely to be incarcerated (Bixby et al., 2022).

According to the Robert Wood Johnson Foundation, "Achieving health equity starts with identifying disparities of concern to stakeholders—particularly those members of affected populations—and their potential causes."[3] To illustrate this, Platt presented on what he described as the "4 Steps to Achieving Health Equity." The first step of health equity includes identifying the upstream social inequities, challenges that affect access to needed resources, and opportunities individuals need to be healthier. The second step of health equity is eliminating the unfair social conditions creating inequity by changing policies, laws, systems, and institutional practices that create barriers and restrict opportunities is critical. While it may take decades or generations to reduce some health disparities, public funders want to see measurable gains

---

[2] C.F.R. §416.926a.

[3] https://www.rwjf.org/en/our-vision/focus-areas/Features/achieving-health-equity.html (accessed June 26, 2024).

BOX 2-3
Key Health Disparities Concepts and Terms

- Health equity: A state of fair and just opportunities to be as healthy as possible (Harper et al., 2010). Equity is both a process and an outcome, often measured as reductions in disparities by improving the health of disadvantaged groups. Achieving health equity requires removing obstacles and increasing opportunities to maximize health, most often by addressing social determinants of health.
- Health disparities: Avoidable, systematic health differences that adversely affect socially (including economically) disadvantaged groups. They are of concern even when their causes are not fully understood because they affect groups already at an underlying disadvantage and may expand the disadvantage with respect to their health.
- Social determinants of health: Nonmedical factors, such as employment, income, housing, transportation, childcare, education, the legal and political system, access to medical care, and the quality of the places people live, work, learn, and play, that influence health and are shaped by social policies (Krieger, 2001).
- Disadvantaged groups: Those who have been excluded from accessing the social and material resources available to other groups in society, often resulting from discrimination or marginalization. These groups include, but are not limited to, people of color, people living in poverty, LGBTQ+ individuals, women, gender-nonconforming individuals, and people with physical and mental disabilities.
- Discrimination: The process by which individuals or groups are treated unfairly because of their perceived or actual group identity as a means of reinforcing positions of power and privilege. Discrimination arises from socially derived beliefs about groups and their members, and it can occur intentionally or unconsciously and be intrapersonal, interpersonal, or structural (Jones, 2000).

SOURCES: Platt presentation, April 4, 2024. Derived from Harper et al., 2010; Krieger, 2001; and Jones, 2000.

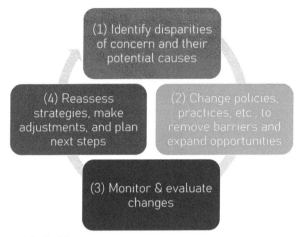

FIGURE 2-3 The health equity process.
SOURCE: Platt presentation, April 4, 2024.

from their investments in the short term too. The third step of health equity is to identify short- and intermediate-term outcome indicators that could be improved within the time frame of an initiative, said Platt.

The fourth step to achieving health equity is to reassess strategies, make adjustments, and plan next steps. "Achieving equity is not a finite project that will be implemented or completed in a predictable period of time," said Platt, explaining:

> It requires a constant process and engaging a cycle of improvement that actively engages those most affected in all stages of the process ... and a sustained commitment to improving health for all, and particularly those with the greatest needs, that must be a deeply held value throughout society.

To end on a hopeful note, Platt discussed successful efforts to reduce social and health inequities. The Villages of East Lake in Atlanta, Georgia, is a community that had experienced a cycle of economic neglect, extreme poverty, violent crime, high unemployment, low educational achievements, and poor health outcomes. A partnership between East Lake residents, the Atlanta Housing Authority, Atlanta Public Schools, and the YMCA created high-quality, mixed-income housing; a cradle-to-college educational pipeline; and wellness resources. This comprehensive community transformation resulted in reduced rates of childhood asthma and obesity, a 90 percent reduction in violent crime, a reduction from 59 to 5 percent of subsidized housing residents on public assistance, and an increase from 13 to 100 percent of nonelderly residents employed or in job training. The success of the East Lake model led to the founding of Purpose

Built Communities, a nonprofit organization that works to replicate the successful elements of the East Lake model in other low-income communities across the nation. Founded in 2009, Purpose Built Communities is now active in 26 communities in 14 states (Purpose Built Communities, 2024).

As an example of a policy that addresses social and health disparities, Platt discussed the 1993 expansion of the earned income tax credit, which gives larger tax refunds to low-income families with children. Studies have shown that expanding the earned income tax credit contributed to improvements in maternal health, mental health, and biological markers of risk for chronic disease (Evans and Garthwaite, 2014). The ADA represents a policy change that expanded access and protections from discrimination for people with disabilities. The Urban Institute's Disability Equity Policy Initiative aims to equip policy makers and practitioners with the rigorous, timely, and actionable research they need to advance economic mobility, housing stability, community connections, and a more accessible and equitable public safety net (Urban Institute, 2024).

THE PURPOSE AND FUNCTION OF THE MEDICAL RECORD

Kensaku Kawamoto explained that the medical record—also called the health record or patient chart—is a record of a patient's medical information, including diagnoses, clinical notes, test results, treatments and procedures, social and family history, and medications. For the most part, the electronic medical record and electronic health record (EHR) are synonymous and contain all the information in a patient's paper chart. In 2004, EHR adoption was at 13 percent; however, the Meaningful Use incentive program has increased EHR adoption to 96 percent of hospitals (ONC, 2021a), and 88 percent of office-based physicians (ONC, 2021b) had adopted EHRs by 2021. Today, most EHRs are commercial systems (Figure 2-4).

Vendor	% Hospitals
Epic*	36%
Oracle Cerner	25%
Meditech	16%
CPSI	8%
Other	15%

Vendor	% Practices
eClinicalWorks	14%
Epic	10%
Athenahealth	8%
NextGen	5%
Other	64%

*Virtually all academic medical centers

FIGURE 2-4 The most commonly used EHR vendor systems.
SOURCES: Kawamoto presentation, slide 4. Data derived from https://www.beckershospitalreview.com/ehrs/ehr-vendor-market-share-in-the-us.html (accessed March 21, 2024); https://www.definitivehc.com/blog/top-ambulatory-ehr-systems (accessed March 21, 2024).

Billing, said Kawamoto, is at the core of EHR systems and is the reason EHRs were first created. Today, they are central to clinical care, quality reporting, and regulatory compliance, serving as accessible repositories of patient information and supporting clinical decision making. In addition, EHRs help automate and streamline clinical workflows and enable standards-based data sharing. Functionality, he added, can differ significantly across EHR systems or even across institutions using the same system because of customizations. While useful, multiple studies have shown that EHRs are a major cause of physician frustration and burnout (Budd, 2023; Calandra et al., 2022; Robertson et al., 2017).

Clinical decision support is an increasingly important EHR function. In this role, an EHR can provide clinicians and patients with knowledge and person-specific information filtered intelligently and presented at appropriate times, such as through alerts and reminders, to enhance health and health care. EHR-based clinical decision support aims to address two research findings: patients, in general, only receive about half of the evidence-based and recommended care, and it takes 15 to 20 years before best practices are adopted widely (National Academy of Medicine, 2017). However, if not done well, decision support can annoy clinicians with too many pop-up alerts.

Kawamoto explained that federal incentives encourage clinicians and hospitals to use certified EHRs. The Office of the National Coordinator for Health Information Technology and the Centers for Medicare & Medicaid Services collaborate to define and regularly update certification requirements. These requirements are the basis for common functionality and interoperability standards applicable to virtually all EHRs. Today, there are penalties for not using a certified EHR. Kawamoto suggested that if SSA would find certain features and information useful, it could make its wishes known to inform future updates to the certification criteria so every EHR could provide the necessary information.

3

Social Determinants of Health and Their Effects on Care

Key Messages from Individual Speakers

- People with a disability (intellectual or developmental) are disadvantaged for almost every indicator of health, whether for physical, oral, or mental health; for risky health behaviors such as smoking and substance use; for chronic health conditions; or for premature mortality. People with a disability who also identify as LGBTQ+ are even more likely to report poor physical and mental health, as are people whose disability affects their mobility, and/or who have minoritized racial and ethnic identities. (Mitra)
- One contributor to the health inequities individuals with disabilities experience is the attitude of physicians and other health care professionals regarding individuals with disabilities. Studies have found that physicians feel uncomfortable, untrained, and unprepared to work with individuals with disabilities. (Mitra)
- The medical record for individuals with disabilities is often incomplete because of the limited time clinicians have to spend with their patients. (Johnson)
- Electronic health records (EHRs) are not providing the information clinicians feel is pertinent for delivering appropriate care to their patients, including having a place to live; having a job and enough resources to provide for their family; having food on the table; and having a sense of purpose, connection, and belonging. (Miller)

- It is important to develop and implement standardized data fields in EHRs for collecting social determinants data, which would allow for consistency and easier analysis and sharing across health systems. (Miller)
- A new rule from the Centers for Medicare & Medicaid Services requiring health care organizations to screen for five social risk drivers is promising, but clinicians need training and technical assistance to enter social determinants into their EHRs. (Hudson)

The workshop's second session introduced the primary social determinants of health and how they affect different populations. This session also discussed challenges and variability in access to care and care delivery, including the potential effects of these health outcomes. The four speakers in this session were Monika Mitra, the Nancy Lurie Marks Professor of Disability Policy and Director of the Lurie Institute for Disability Policy at Brandeis University; Joy Amaryllis Johnson, resident services coordinator with the Charlottesville Redevelopment and Housing Authority and a disability advocate; Benjamin F. Miller, a clinical psychologist and adjunct faculty at Stanford School of Medicine; and Jennifer Hudson, developmental director at the Williamson Health and Wellness Center. Ruqaiijah Yearby, planning committee member and the Kara J. Trott Professor in Health Law at the Ohio State University Moritz College of Law, moderated a question-and-answer period following the four presentations.

ADDRESSING SOCIAL DETERMINANTS OF HEALTH FOR PEOPLE WITH DISABILITIES

Monika Mitra said people with a disability are disadvantaged for almost every indicator of health, whether for physical, oral, or mental health; for risky health behaviors such as smoking and substance use; for chronic health conditions; or for premature mortality. She noted that people with a disability who also identify as LGBTQ+ are even more likely to report poor physical and mental health, as are people with an intellectual or developmental disability or whose disability affects their mobility and who have minoritized racial and ethnic identities (Mitra et al., 2022).

Much of Mitra's research has focused on pregnancy, perinatal health, and reproductive health, and her studies have found that pregnant women with disabilities are at a significant disadvantage regarding pregnancy complications, access to prenatal care, adverse outcomes, postpartum health, and perinatal mental health. For example, pregnant women with intellectual and developmental disabilities have a 75 percent higher risk for severe maternal morbidity and a 186 percent higher risk for maternal mortality compared to peers without an intellectual or developmental disability (Mitra et al., 2021). Women who are deaf or hard of hearing have an 80 percent higher risk for severe maternal morbidity (Mitra et al., 2024).

Mitra said the intersection between disability and health is rarely part of policy or programmatic discussions, which she believes stems from the expectations that people with disabilities will have poor health because of their disabilities. In reality, she said, health disparities and health inequities resulting from social determinants of health cause the poor health people with disabilities experience (see Box 3-1). Social determinants of health refer to the conditions in which people are born, grow, live, work, and age, as well as the wider set of forces and systems shaping the conditions of daily life. These social determinants include factors such as socioeconomic status, education, neighborhood and physical environment, employment, social support networks, access to health care, and access to resources such as food and transportation.

In particular, said Mitra, some social determinants of health have unique effects on the health, well-being, and quality of life of people with disabilities, including:

BOX 3-1
Health Disparity, Health Care Disparity,
Health Inequality, and Health Inequity

- Health disparities are differences in health and well-being outcomes without an identified cause among groups of people.
- Health care disparities are differences in the quality of health care received that do not result from access-related factors or clinical needs, preferences, or intervention appropriateness.
- Health inequalities are differences in health status or in the distribution of health determinants among different population groups, such as the differences in mobility between older and younger populations or in mortality rates between people from different social classes.
- Health inequities are differences in health and well-being outcomes that are avoidable, unfair, and unjust and that are affected by social, economic, and environmental conditions.

SOURCES: Mitra presentation, April 4, 2024, and Gómez et al., 2021.

- restricted environmental access,
- the pejorative and stigmatizing attitudes of health care providers,
- the administrative burden associated with complex procedures and policies that disabled people often experience when interacting with the social systems around them,
- the lack of social supports and systems, and
- the lack of home supports and community-based supports that would enable people with disabilities to live in the community rather than in institutional settings.

Mitra noted the vast differences in educational attainment, particularly for postsecondary education, between people with and without a disability. Only 2 percent of students with intellectual disabilities receive any college education because of low expectations and a lack of emphasis and inclusion of people with intellectual disabilities in higher education. People with any disability are less likely to work compared to people with no disability, and people with a cognitive disability are the least likely to work (Winsor et al., 2023). The poverty rate among people with a disability is more than twice that of those without a disability.

Mitra explained that people with disabilities pay a "disability tax," the extra financial burdens that individuals with disabilities often face because of the additional costs associated with their condition, including expenses for specialized medical care, assistive devices, modifications to living spaces or vehicles for accessibility, transportation, personal care assistance, and other accommodations necessary for daily living. When accounting for this disability tax, the rate of disabled people living in poverty is approximately 35 percent. On average, she added, a household with a member with a disability requires 29 percent more income to obtain a comparable standard of living to a household without disabled members (Morris et al. 2021).

Given their lower employment rates and higher rates of poverty, individuals with a disability have significantly higher rates of food insecurity and housing insecurity (Coleman-Jensen, 2020; Meschede et al., 2023). The affordable housing crisis, said Mitra, has a significant effect on people with disabilities who need accessible housing so they can live in the community. Supplemental Security Income (SSI), for example, does not cover the average rent for a studio or one-bedroom apartment in any housing market across the United States (TAC, 2014). On average, households with members with any type of disability live in poorer quality housing and neighborhoods.

Transportation is another social determinant of health that people with disabilities deal with regularly. Transportation barriers can present significant challenges for individuals with disabilities, limiting their ability to access essential services, employment opportunities, social activities, and health care.

In many parts of the country, accessible public transportation and paratransit services are limited or unavailable. People with blindness or low vision, psychiatric disabilities, chronic health conditions, or multiple disabilities experience more problems using public transportation, Mitra added (Bezyak et al., 2020). Regarding social networks and social isolation, Mitra said data from her team show that people with a disability who identify as belonging to a sexual orientation or gender identity minority are at a great disadvantage.

One contributor to the health inequities individuals with disabilities experience is the attitude of physicians and other health care professionals regarding individuals with disabilities. Studies have found that physicians feel uncomfortable, untrained, and unprepared to work with individuals with disabilities. According to Mitra, 81 percent of medical students and 75 percent of residents have no clinical training in disability care (Holder et al., 2009). One study from her group found that 44 percent of obstetrics/gynecology clinics in four cities reported being unable to provide care for people with mobility disabilities (Mitra et al., 2016). When questioned about the quality of life of people with disabilities, 82.4 percent of clinicians said they expected quality of life to be "a little" or "a lot" worse. In the same survey, only 56.5 percent of clinicians strongly agreed with the statement, "I welcome patients with a disability into my practice," and only 40.7 percent were "very confident" they could provide the same quality of care to patients with or without a disability (Iezzoni et al., 2021).

Mitra said health disparities and inequities cannot be treated in a vacuum of health care. She noted that in 2023, the National Institutes of Health designated people with disabilities as a population with health disparities (NIH, 2023). She hopes this announcement will lead to a larger body of work aimed at documenting and understanding the disparities and the upstream and downstream factors evidence-based programs need to address to support individuals with disabilities.

PERSPECTIVE OF A COMMUNITY
OUTREACH COORDINATOR

To provide some context for her remarks, Joy Amaryllis Johnson said she has a grandson with a neurodevelopmental disability who has had his disability application denied because his mother makes too much money as an ultrasound technician. She also has a daughter who lost part of her leg in a work accident and whose disability application has been denied six times. Johnson, who characterized herself as being morbidly obese, has found physicians to be disrespectful and dismissive when she tries to find solutions to her obesity. Johnson said, in her role as a community outreach coordinator, she takes on a great deal of trauma while trying to assist individuals in her community who have a disability. She noted, too, that the medical record for individuals with disabilities is often incomplete because of the limited time clinicians have to spend with their patients.

Johnson, who works on public housing and welcoming people into the community, said too many developers think only about their bottom line and not about how to make their buildings compliant with requirements in the Americans with Disabilities Act (ADA). "Nobody is holding developers or agencies accountable for this," said Johnson. "Every unit we build should be ADA compliant."

REIMAGINING EHRs TO INCLUDE THE SOCIAL SIDE OF HEALTH

"Understanding and addressing the social determinants [of health] is paramount for effectively addressing mental health. Full stop," said Benjamin F. Miller at the start of his presentation. Research, he said, consistently shows this interplay between social factors—socioeconomic status, access to education, employment, and others—and mental health. These determinants not only influence an individual's susceptibility to mental health disorders, but also affect access to treatment, recovery, outcomes, and well-being. "By recognizing and addressing these connections and seeing them as a core component of what we do in practice, we actually are able to better address issues like mental health and society as a whole," said Miller.

The era of electronic health records (EHRs) began on a note of optimism, but the way EHRs have affected systems and workflows differs significantly from the original intent of the EHR, he said. The vision for EHRs was that they would enhance communication and improve recordkeeping; based on recent data, it is still unclear whether EHRs deliver any efficiencies. "What we know is our system has become skewed towards clicks or data entry that represents a complete task within EHRs," said Miller, a trend he blamed for the relationship between EHR use and physician burnout. Studies have shown, for example, that providers who spend more than six hours a week outside of normal clinic hours completing EHRs were nearly three times more likely to report burnout overall and almost four times more likely to say that EHRs themselves were the major cause of their burnout (Robertson et al., 2017).

EHRs, said Miller, are not providing the information clinicians feel is pertinent for delivering appropriate care to their patients. "In 2024, it really feels time to refocus our EHRs to serve not just as documentation tools but as instruments for a more comprehensive and community orientation approach to well-being," said Miller. Individuals in certain communities, he noted, bear a disproportionate burden of population health psychiatric morbidity. "Given that poor mental health can significantly hinder life expectancy and the quality of it, it underscores the importance of prioritizing population mental health that includes addressing social determinants," said Miller.

When researchers ask people what matters most to them and their health, the answers are invariably having a place to live; having a job and enough resources to provide for their family; having food on the table; and having a sense of purpose, connection, and belonging. These conditions, said Miller, are vital conditions, yet EHRs track few if any of these conditions, even when clinicians ask about them. Specific to mental health, these vital conditions represent some of the most modifiable intervention targets, but the complexity of the U.S. health care system makes it difficult to reformulate how to tackle massive issues such as the social determinants of health and mental health.

The mental health field, unlike other branches of health care, has done less to embrace preventive approaches and has less grounding in prevention than other areas of medicine, said Miller. "For mental health, most of our resources have been devoted to secondary and tertiary treatment of existing mental health disorders versus actually preventing them in the first place," he said. "The inability of the mental health field to work upstream and prevent poor mental health hinders progress in reducing the incidence, prevalence, and burden of mental health disorders."

Miller discussed several key challenges around workflow, technology, incentives, and privacy that need addressing to collect and use data on the social determinants of health in clinical settings. He acknowledged that getting people to change the way they do things is difficult, as anyone who has engaged in health care transformation has experienced. Getting clinicians to change their practices requires support and technical assistance. Regarding data on the social determinants, it is important to make the data relevant to providers and to incorporate data collection into workflows in a manner that does not disrupt their day. Otherwise, said Miller, clinicians will see this as yet another unfunded mandate handed down from administration.

Regarding data, Miller said it is important to develop and implement standardized data fields in EHRs for collecting social determinants data, which would allow for consistency and easier analysis and sharing across health systems. Efforts to extract data on mental health from EHRs have fared poorly because those data are not consistently structured across multiple EHRs. He does not want to see this happen for the social determinants.

Getting clinicians to collect data on social determinants will require payment systems to change their payment policies. In the current health care payment systems, clinicians get paid for procedures performed, not for time spent collecting social determinants data. Today, there are not enough incentives to move the needle on data collection, though holding systems accountable for either collecting those data or using them in a meaningful way would lead to progress. Miller noted there are technology tools for bringing social determinants into EHRs. One place to start, he said, is to use natural language processing tools to automatically extract social determinants data from clinical notes. This would reduce the burden on clinicians and ensure data are captured and studied in a meaningful way.

Miller said the most expensive mental health services are those used the least (Figure 3-1). However, he added, "We do little to put resources into the bottom of the pyramid." As an example, he recounted a study he and his colleagues conducted that looked at how much California spent on health care versus social programs. "What we found is likely the case throughout all states, with this disturbing paradox where increased state spending on medical treatment may actually contribute to worse health conditions because of ignoring the investment on the social side of health," said Miller. Limited budgets and siloed funding are significant barriers to changing the ratio of spending on health care versus social determinants of health.

What matters most going forward, said Miller, is the need to be intentional about investments and policies that promote social determinants as being foundations for health. Because the public is more aware today of how social factors affect their health, this may be the moment to act and enable EHRs to collect these data.

Miller shared a cautionary tale related to integrating mental health into primary care. Numerous studies show the benefits of bringing mental health clinicians into primary care (Gallo and Barlow, 2012; O'Loughlin et al., 2019; Rowan et al., 2021), yet adoption has been slow, at least in part because the

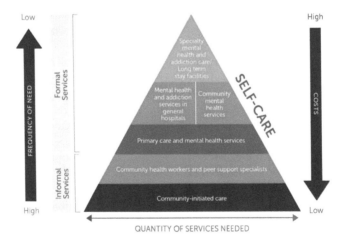

FIGURE 3-1 The inverse relationship between the most used behavioral health services and cost.
SOURCES: Miller presentation, April 4, 2024. Modified from World Health Organization (WHO). 2009. CC-BY-NC-SA 3.0.

incentives have been too low and too easy to achieve and because too many clinicians are not aware of the value of doing so. Miller said:

> If we are serious about bringing social determinants into health care and incorporating them into EHRs, we have to make it matter for those on the frontline. Make it easy for them. Help them to see the value and then wrap that up through meaningful support.

Incorporating social determinants into EHRs, said Miller, will provide a more complete picture of patient health and enable health care providers to better address mental health and the root causes of health disparities. "Taking a more comprehensive approach to health really allows a more intentional and meaningful way to achieve positive outcomes for all populations," he said in closing.

AN INTEGRATED AND PATIENT-CENTERED CARE MODEL

Jennifer Hudson explained that her health center's network serves as a convener to bring together social services partners and assist with bringing together resources to support healthy eating, active living, transportation, mental well-being, and social connections in the community. She noted that rural Williamson, West Virginia, where she works, is among the most impoverished communities in the United States. It is also an area with some of the highest rates in the country of chronic diseases, such as diabetes and heart disease. Adults with disabilities in West Virginia experience health disparities; are more likely to have depression, obesity, diabetes, and heart disease; and are more likely to smoke. Nearly 36 percent of adults in West Virginia have a disability. She added that while good things are happening in this community, the publicly available data do not reflect that yet.

In 2024, a new rule from the Centers for Medicare & Medicaid Services (CMS) uses new payment models to encourage health care organizations to perform more services aimed at addressing social determinants of health. This rule by CMS only affects patients who have Medicare, but it paves the way for change with other insurance payers who may also introduce billing codes that cover these types of services in the future. Hudson believes the new rule is promising, but clinicians need training and technical assistance to enter social determinants into their EHRs. When pulling meaningful information from the EHR, developing a structured report is expensive, as is buying a new platform that sits on top of the medical record to extract information from the data.

Q&A WITH THE PANELISTS

Ruqaiijah Yearby began the discussion by noting how difficult it has been to get clinicians to include data on the social determinants in the EHR. It may be necessary, she said, to expand the process to include statements from individuals and community health workers to consider how the social determinants of health can affect that process.

Yearby asked Johnson to talk about how housing, equity, and access to health care are connected. Housing is a human right, replied Johnson, and without housing an individual's health probably will not be the best. She noted that most of her organization's clients have chronic disabilities, and their need is for an efficiency apartment, not a two-bedroom unit. However, developers are not building efficiencies. She advocates for these disabled individuals when meeting with funders, developers, and the Charlottesville Redevelopment and Housing Authority and reminds them of the need to comply with the rules of the Americans with Disabilities Act.

Michael V. Stanton, a licensed clinical health psychologist and associate professor of public health at California State University, East Bay, asked the panelists to discuss how mental health challenges can create difficulties for people to receive benefits. Johnson replied there are statutes and policies that contribute to this problem and that need to change. Miller said another contributor is that people with a mental illness are seen as a relatively homogenous population defined by their diagnosis. However, some individuals with a mental health issue are highly functional and have no impairment in their daily lives, while others with a mild or moderate diagnosis are severely impaired. They are also frequently codified into one population, which makes treating each individual effectively more difficult. This dichotomous view— one either does or does not have a mental illness—hinders taking a more all-encompassing view of how mental health is foundational to health and an individual's ability to address social determinants and improve their mental health.

A second issue, said Miller, is that the nation has reinforced faulty structures that lead to the idea that mental health is separate from physical health. Today, however, mental health has garnered public attention, making it an ideal time to create new structures that bring care to where people are and break down the silos that separate mental and physical health. "That, to me, is the future and the only way we are going to make meaningful progress in this space," said Miller.

4

Disparities and Bias in Evaluative Testing and Recording of Medical Information

Key Messages from Individual Speakers

- Ensuring fairness in artificial intelligence (AI) applications is necessary for advancing health equity, and that depends on selecting the appropriate data for training an algorithm, how the algorithm is designed, and how it is deployed in clinics and hospitals. (Chin)
- Individuals and organizations must accept responsibility and be accountable for achieving equity and fairness in outcomes from health care algorithms. (Chin)
- There are areas of the application for disability determination that fall short of being inclusive. The level of documentation required can be troubling for anybody of any race, but that documentation is difficult to obtain for minoritized individuals because of the difficulty they have getting a diagnosis. (Thornton)
- A survey of physicians across the country found that only 60 percent would welcome people with disabilities in their practices, only 40 percent were very confident in their ability to provide quality care, and 36 percent knew little to nothing about the Americans with Disabilities Act. (Lagu)
- There is no federal law and few state mandates, as there is with race and ethnicity, to collect data on disability, and as a result, there are limited data on how many people with disabilities do not get recommended health care interventions. (Lagu)

- Being diagnosed with a disability can put a target on one's back and can cause more oppression and more people to treat an individual with a disability differently. (Link)
- In Black communities, parents, caregivers, and community members want to protect people from being labeled by medical professionals as disabled. As a result, they do not interact with the health care system for fear that being labeled as having a disability will cause more structural harms. This leads to underrepresentation of Black individuals in some disability datasets. (Link)

The workshop's third session discussed common tests and clinical algorithms that are inaccurate or inappropriate for specific populations, inequities in accessing diagnostic testing and treatment that may negatively affect disability applications, and biases in the documentation of clinicians of care in the medical record and how findings from tests or screens deemed as objective medical evidence may be minimized. The four speakers in this session were Marshall H. Chin, the Richard Parrillo Family distinguished service professor of health care ethics at the University of Chicago; Gloria Thornton, founder of Amplified Disabled Voices LLC; Tara Lagu, professor of medicine and medical social sciences and the director of the Center for Health Services and Outcomes Research at the Northwestern University Feinberg School of Medicine; and AJ Link, president of the National Disabled Legal Professionals Association and an adjunct professor of space law at Howard University School of Law. Rupa Valdez, planning committee member and professor at the University of Virginia and president of the Blue Trunk Foundation, moderated a brief question-and-answer period following the four presentations.

GUIDING PRINCIPLES TO ADDRESS THE EFFECT OF ALGORITHM BIAS ON DISPARITIES IN HEALTH AND HEALTH CARE

Marshall H. Chin said a paper he and his colleagues published in 2023 on how to address algorithmic bias received a great deal of attention, including from the White House, because it pertains to actions regarding the way artificial intelligence (AI) uses algorithms (Chin et al., 2023). He explained that a health care algorithm is a mathematical model used to inform decision making, such as determining whether someone has a disability or not. An algorithm could also be used for treatment, prognosis, risk stratification, triage, and the allocation of resources. AI, he explained, learns by inferring relationships in a large dataset. The issue is that an algorithm is a black box with limited transparency for how it produces its results.

An unbiased algorithm, said Chin, is one in which patients with the same algorithm score or classification have the same basic needs. An example of a biased algorithm is one clinicians have used to determine who is eligible for a kidney transplant. This algorithm inaccurately assigned higher levels of kidney function to Black patients compared to White patients with the same score on glomerular filtration rate, a primary measure of kidney function. This flaw resulted in delays in referral for kidney transplant for Black individuals (Vyas et al., 2020). Perhaps the most famous example examined a proprietary commercial algorithm designed to determine who would be eligible for chronic disease management programs (Obermeyer et al., 2019). This algorithm made it such that Black patients had to be sicker than White patients to qualify for these programs because it used money and resource use as a proxy for health.

Chin explained that biases can arise in both model development and use. The algorithm that powers pulse oximetry, for example, overestimates oxygen saturation in Black individuals (Shi et al., 2022). Ensuring fairness in AI applications is necessary for advancing health equity, he said, and that depends on selecting the appropriate data for training an algorithm, how the algorithm is designed, and how it is deployed in clinics and hospitals (Rajkomar et al., 2018).

In response to a request from Congress, Chin cochaired a nine-person diverse panel to develop five guiding principles to address the effect of health care algorithms on racial and ethnic inequities in health and health care, each of which is operationalized at the individual, institutional, and societal levels (Figure 4-1). While many groups developing algorithms start with data selection, Chin argued that determining the problem at hand before thinking about data is critical, particularly if the algorithm's goal is to maximize the health of patients and communities. "In some ways, if you have the wrong problem and goal, that is just the setup for all types of bad things happening," said Chin. Also important is looking for bias at each of the different phases of an algorithm's life cycle.

The first guiding principle is to promote equity in all phases of an algorithm's life cycle. Health equity, said Chin, means that everyone has a fair and just opportunity to be healthy. Achieving health equity requires valuing everyone equally, with focused and ongoing societal efforts to address avoidable inequalities, as well as historical and contemporary injustices, which includes addressing systemic racism and the elimination of health and health care disparities. A fair and equitable algorithm produces equitable outcomes.

The second guiding principle—ensure transparency and explainability— means that all relevant individuals should understand how their data are used

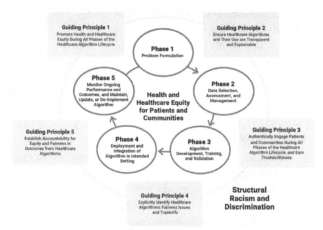

FIGURE 4-1 Guiding principles and the algorithm life cycle.
SOURCES: Chin presentation, April 4, 2024; Chin et al., 2023. CC-BY-NC-ND.

and how AI systems make decisions. To be transparent, every algorithm, its attributions and its correlations, should be open to inspection. Explanations should correctly reflect the system's process for generating output, which should be used only when the system achieves sufficient confidence in its results (Zuckerman et al., 2022).

Chin said the third principle is to authentically engage patients and communities to earn trust. This requires engaging patients in choosing a problem, selecting the data to inform the algorithm, developing and deploying the algorithm, and monitoring its output. "Patients must know how an algorithm affects their care," he said. Trustworthiness, he added, is earned through authenticity, ethical practices, data security, and timely disclosures of algorithm use. He noted there are important data sovereignty issues for American Indians and Alaska Natives regarding data ownership.

The fourth principle—identify fairness issues and trade-offs—is critical, said Chin. Algorithmic fairness and bias issues arise from both ethical choices and technical decisions at each stage of the algorithm's life cycle. It is important to identify fairness and bias issues and address them directly, with fair distribution of social benefit and burden serving as an ethical framework for judging fairness and bias. From a technical perspective, Chin explained that different technical definitions of algorithmic fairness are mathematically mutually incompatible, trading off maximizing accuracy of an algorithm for entire groups and minimizing accuracy differences among subgroups across definitions.

The panel's report argues for mitigating bias both through social means, by having diverse teams and codevelopment, and by using technical algorithmic fairness tool kits. "We also need to view algorithms and accompanying policies and regulations through frames of equity of harms and risks," said Chin, particularly for algorithms dealing with disability where there is the potential for high-risk and high-harm issues to arise. Models, said Chin, should be optimized for equity in clinical outcomes or resource allocation using bias mitigation methods and human judgment, with explicit identification of trade-offs among competing values and options.

The final principle is accountability. Individuals and organizations must accept responsibility and be accountable for achieving equity and fairness in outcomes from health care algorithms. Organizations should be comprehensive in establishing processes at each stage of the life cycle of the algorithm to facilitate equity and fairness in outcomes. Organizations should also have an inventory of their algorithms and periodically screen them for, and mitigate, bias. Chin said:

> We think it is important to have very important oversight of prediction models, with checkpoint gates at each phase of the algorithm life cycle, oversight governance structures that involve the public, and an investment in the infrastructure to do things the right way in terms of avoiding bias.

All regulations and incentives should support equity and fairness, and algorithms should not be deployed before validating them on the affected population. In addition, "those persons and communities who have been harmed by unfair algorithms should be redressed," said Chin.

Chin concluded his presentation with a list of overarching issues and challenges:

- Technical definitions and metrics of fairness rarely translate clearly or intuitively to ethical, legal, social, and economic conceptions of fairness.
- Trade-offs among competing fairness metrics and values are common.
- There is no cookie-cutter solution to fairness and equity, making it imperative to individualize each use case.
- There can be trade-offs between equity and justice versus efficiency and saving money.
- Communication challenges include explaining probabilities and distributions, assessing and explaining real data and synthetic data, assessing and explaining the validity of applying a specific algorithm to a specific individual, and explaining the difference between legal informed consent and patients truly understanding and providing informed consent.

Regulations and incentives, said Chin, should support equity and fairness while also promoting innovation. In addition, the AI field needs to create an ethical, legal, social, and administrative framework and culture that redresses harm while encouraging quality improvement, collaboration, and transparency similar to recommendations for patient safety. As a final comment, he said,

> ChatGPT and other AI language models have spurred widespread public interest in the potential value and dangers of algorithms. Multiple stakeholders must partner to create systems, processes, regulations, incentives, standards, and policies to mitigate and prevent algorithm bias in health care. Dedicated resources and the support of leaders and the public are critical for successful reform. It is our obligation to avoid repeating errors that tainted use of algorithms in other fields.

HEALTH INEQUITIES THROUGH THE LENS
OF A PERSON WITH DISABILITIES

Gloria Thornton said that as a person with disabilities, she has been treated in a variety of ways, and she noticed that multiple factors contribute to why she is treated differently, including being a woman, being African American, having invisible disabilities, being visibly disabled, having a mental health diagnosis, and being educated. "Whenever I speak on this topic, it is coming from a place of passion and love, but also frustration and a level of sadness," she said.

When Thornton was in middle school, she began having noticeable health issues that doctors kept dismissing as anxiety, depression, a lack of social skills, or a failure to thrive. "This is when my fear of medical providers started and my medical files began to receive life-altering notes that made finding reputable doctors for my care difficult," she explained.

In December 2020, Thornton contracted aseptic meningitis from a treatment one of her most trusted clinicians suggested via home health. "While the doctor was amazing, the nurse that I had at the time decided that my doctor's instructions were too long, and she did not want to stay at my house for the allotted twelve hours, so she did the twelve-hour treatment in four," said Thornton. The result was an almost two-week stay in the hospital, where she had time to think about what happened to her and experience of medical biases firsthand. Because of the emergence of COVID-19 at that time, she was sent home prematurely but had to be readmitted several days later. During this admission, the doctor on her floor refused her multiple daily medications and pain medications, although he could see her visible pain. His reason was that "People like you don't have pain from diseases like this."

In July 2022, Thornton was experiencing back pain and saw a physician assistant who told her he would help her find answers. However, after ordering a couple of tests, he sent her a note telling her to find someone else because her problems were "above his pay grade." "Stories like this are all too common," said Thornton, who added that having information in the EHR that paints an individual as being noncompliant, incompetent, lying, or exaggerating will lead to many adversities in getting care. For one thing, it was difficult for her to get assistance through either Social Security Disability Insurance (SSDI) or Supplemental Security Income (SSI). "This is why it is important to focus on specific definitions of terms used within different health records and program requirements," she said.

According to federal regulations, the law defines disability, for the purpose of Social Security disability programs for adults, as the inability to do any substantial gainful activity for any medically determinable physical or mental impairment that will likely result in death or that has lasted or will likely last for a continuous period of not less than twelve months. While this definition sounds simple and unbiased, there are areas of the application for disability determination that fall short of being inclusive, said Thornton. The level of documentation required can be troubling for anybody of any race, but that documentation is difficult to obtain for minoritized individuals because of the difficulty they have getting a diagnosis. Thornton was told by the hospital system that her records had been destroyed or did not exist. "As a minority disabled woman, I often believe sometimes I am better off avoiding doctors and medical offices due to the amount of medical biases, discrepancies, and ableism I endured," she said. In the end, she retracted her application,

After describing the multiple steps and multiple clinicians that must be involved to receive a new wheelchair, Thornton said she works as an ombudsman for others to address the problems that create delays. "As an advocate, I use my voice to speak for people with disabilities who are unable to receive the items they need in order to receive the best care," she said. As a final comment, she noted that SSI and SSDI are designed to help people with disabilities, but the process is so tedious that people like herself either start the application and do not complete it or they attempt to complete the application, receive a denial, and do not try again. "The policies surrounding SSDI and SSI and the definition of disability need to be reassessed in order to focus on the population being helped," said Thornton. "This is a process designed to help people, but instead it results in people with disabilities dealing with the consistent stress of [getting] approval."

DATA COLLECTION AND IDENTIFICATION OF DISABILITY STATUS: NECESSARY TOOLS TO IMPROVE CARE ACCESS AND REDUCE HEALTH CARE DISPARITIES FOR PEOPLE WITH DISABILITIES

Tara Lagu recalled how when she was discharging a patient who used a wheelchair, she could not get her an appointment with a subspecialist, and as she rolled out the door, the patient said this was discrimination. Thinking this assessment was correct, Lagu spent the next year calling subspecialists around the country and asked them if they would make an appointment for a fictional patient who used a wheelchair. What she found was shocking: approximately 22 percent of the 256 practices she contacted would not make an appointment for someone in a wheelchair, either because their practices were in inaccessible buildings or because they could not transfer the patient to an exam table. Slightly more than half of the other clinicians planned to transfer the patient to the exam table manually, which is considered dangerous, and less than 10 percent of the practices had adjustable tables or other accessible equipment.

After publishing her findings (Lagu et al., 2013), Lagu began looking into how this major inequity existed when legislation protects the rights of people with disabilities. "It seems there are persistent disparities in health care access for this group of people," she said. With two colleagues, she wrote a paper describing what clinicians should do in three realms to care for people with disabilities: physical access, communication access, and programmatic access (Lagu et al., 2014). Enabling physical access requires having room next to the exam table for a wheelchair, an adjustable height table, space to allow transfers, and an accessible route in and out of the exam room.

Communication access means that providers and patients should work together to identify alternative communication methods for patients with disabilities, whether that be having telecommunication devices or sign language interpreters for people with hearing loss, or large print forms for individuals with visual impairments. Programmatic access requires universal access to scheduling, staffing, and other administrative resources; that the system alerts the receptionist and staff when a patient with a disability makes an appointment; and that a room with an accessible table is reserved for the patient's appointment. When she gets pushback on the need for the scheduling system to alert staff, she counters by pointing out that people with a penicillin allergy rarely get penicillin because that information is in the EHR.

Though Lagu and her colleagues published their second paper in the *New England Journal of Medicine*, nothing has changed. A subsequent study of clinics with or without adjustable tables found that individuals with disabilities receiving care in those clinics with height adjustable tables reported no difference in perceived quality of care or the exam they received (Morris et al., 2017). This finding suggested the problem may be related to physician attitudes, so Lagu and colleagues surveyed 71 physicians across the country and found that only 56.5 percent would welcome people with disabilities in their practices, only 40 percent were very confident in their ability to provide quality care, and 36 percent knew little to nothing about the Americans with Disabilities Act of 1990 (ADA) (Iezzoni et al., 2021, 2022).

Speaking with clinicians in focus groups, she found many of the same barriers (Lagu et al., 2022). In addition, some clinicians described specific strategies they use to discharge people with disabilities from their practices. One reason the clinicians gave was that they do not want to fill out the paperwork required for SSDI or SSI. "If you think about this, the need to document medical issues for the Social Security Administration (SSA) is not possible if you cannot get an appointment with a doctor or if your doctor discharges you from their practice," said Lagu. "This might explain some of the disparities in health care access and quality we have seen." This, she added, is the ableism that exists in the nation's health care system and is keeping people with disabilities from getting the care they need and the documentation they need to get the services and benefits SSA can offer.

Lagu noted there is limited federal law and few state mandates, as there is with race and ethnicity, to collect data on disability. As a result, there are no data on how many people with disabilities do not get cancer screenings or cardiovascular interventions. While some health systems want to collect these data, they are discouraged from doing so because if they collect the data and the data reveal gaps in care and a failure to provide the needed accommodations, they will be at risk of unfavorable comparisons to peer organizations that do not collect these data. Without a mandate, few health systems will collect the data voluntarily for all patients, said Lagu, pointing to the need for federal or state laws, policies, and procedures requiring data collection. There is also the need, she added, to incorporate collecting data on disability status into hospital and health system accreditation criteria.

Another issue, said Lagu, is the confusion arising from varying definitions of disability, which raises the question of why the SSA and ADA definitions differ. Lagu explained the ADA is civil rights law, and civil rights should be inclusive and broad, while SSA needs to limit the number of eligible beneficiaries. Complicating the matter, health systems might be on board with collecting the information to accommodate patients, bridging gaps in care, and not violating the ADA, but they are less interested in sharing data from their EHRs if it is used to determine disability, fearing that third parties will use the data for reasons that are beyond the scope of medical care.

A third issue is that prior attempts to identify disability from the EHR alone have failed, and a fourth issue is the lack of standard questions about disability and accommodations, making data collection challenging. Existing questions from the Department of Health and Human Services (HHS) are broad and do not accurately capture disability severity or chronicity (Figure 4-2). In addition, there are no validated questions about accommodations and no support to conduct the research to validate such questions.

There is also unclear buy-in from the National Institutes of Health (NIH) and other federal agencies where people with disabilities experience disparities. Lagu noted that the Centers for Disease Control and Prevention, HHS, the Agency for Healthcare Research and Quality, and NIH now recognize disability as a disparity population, but she is waiting to see if these federal organizations will take the necessary steps to support data collection or fund studies that focus on disability independent of race and other social vulnerabilities.

To remedy this situation, Lagu called for working with advocacy groups to highlight and, when possible, address these structural barriers and encouraged being outspoken about these issues. Health systems, EHR vendors, and insurance companies are not the enemy, she added. "I have found that health systems, vendors, and insurance companies actually want to work with us, but they also want the mandate from federal and state governments," she said. She noted that she is doing research on the margins, so some of this work will get done, but some will not because it will not get funded.

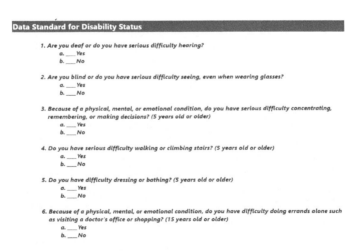

FIGURE 4-2 Standard data HHS collects on disability.
SOURCES: Lagu presentation, April 4, 2024; https://minorityhealth.hhs.gov/omh/browse.aspx?lvl=3&lvlid=53 (accessed February 2024).

BARRIERS TO INITIATE PARTICIPATION IN
INTERACTING WITH THE SYSTEM

AJ Link told the workshop he is openly autistic, a nonapparent disability, and has other identities, such as being a Black man from Florida, a southerner, a new husband, and a father. "Those are all identities that I carry around the world with me, but that also impacts how I experience going through the health care system when I decide to do it and have the autonomy to choose that," said Link. He added that he has a different experience than many people with autism because he was diagnosed as an adult and has good health insurance. For him, it was empowering to learn he is autistic because it explained why he struggled with so many things. Although his diagnosis was a powerful revelation for him, Link said that is not always true, particularly for people from marginalized backgrounds. "Oftentimes, being diagnosed can put a target on your back. It can cause more oppression and cause more people to treat you differently," he said.

Link discussed the barriers to getting care in historically marginalized communities. There is a stigma attached to being disabled, especially if the disability is not apparent. This is especially true for school, where special education was created to reinforce racism and segregation (Connor and Ferri, 2005). In Black communities, he said, patients, caregivers, and community members want to protect people from being labeled as disabled, so they do not interact with the health care system for fear that being labeled as having a disability will cause more structural harms.

Financial issues can be another barrier, and not just being able to afford the cost of a health care visit. Taking time from work, taking the time to find the right physician to see, and having to take public transportation to get to an appointment are the kinds of barriers that prevent people in historically marginalized communities from seeking care. Quality of care is another issue, said Link. "We all know the structural inequalities in our society and where the best care is available," he said, referring to the geographic barriers to accessing quality care.

The health care system itself and the history of medical racism and abuses the Black community has experienced are other barriers to seeking care, said Link. He also noted the benefits of classism and who benefits from being labeled as disabled. "There is racism within the disabled community, but there is also a level of classism," said Link. "Most people who are fortunate enough to openly identify as disabled like I am come from a higher stratum of class, where they are protected from the discrimination, the stigma, and then the consequences of being openly disabled."

Link noted that from a medical perspective, the discussion can center on diagnoses, prescriptions, and recommendations, but regarding adequate access to care, there is the issue of overcoming historical mistrust and convincing people they will receive quality care that will be helpful. He also questioned whether information about quality care is accessible to marginalized communities in nonmedicalized language.

Another challenge is educating marginalized communities about the benefits available to people with disabilities, such as SSDI or SSI, and the protections they have under civil rights laws such as the ADA or the Rehabilitation Act of 1973. Link asked:

> How are we providing that social education that shows that you can use a disabled diagnosis or a diagnosis of a disability as an opportunity to fight for your equal rights when it comes to things like housing, when it comes to things like education, when it comes to things like protection?

Finally, there is the cultural aspect to accessing care. "How do we provide support for those communities that want to be more accessible but do not want to interact with a system that is incredibly racist and ableist?" he asked. "How do we provide the tools for communities to self-accommodate and to identify some of the consequences of disability?" There is a balance here between self-accommodation and seeking care for impairments that need attention from a medical professional. The answer to that problem is to empower people to understand the different disabilities that need medical intervention and disabilities that are strictly problematic because of ableist systems within our communities, he said.

Q&A WITH THE PANELISTS

Rupa Valdez opened the discussion by asking Chin to provide examples of tests or procedures that are less accurate for certain population subgroups. Chin explained that clinical tests often have a normal range, and the question is, where do these normal values originate and how are they adjusted for a patient's race? Many times, he said, these adjustments are "basically voodoo" and result from explicitly racist attitudes. For example, the racial adjustments for a pulmonary function test were based on a mistaken nineteenth-century view that Black people had less ability to metabolize oxygen and had less lung capacity. The problem, he said, arises when the medical community blindly accepts these reference values even though the scientific evidence base for them is faulty. At the same time, changing a reference value can have downstream effects for determining disability eligibility, so there needs to be the evidence base to make that change. "We cannot divorce some of these technical questions from the societal issues that are involved," said Chin. For that reason, it is imperative to involve the affected communities, be transparent and explicit about identifying ethical issues, and then address them rather than "sweeping them under the rug."

Valdez asked the panelists to comment on how identifying biased or untrustworthy health care providers changes how people with disabilities seek care. Link replied that it stops people from seeking care that could be beneficial or even lifesaving, and people choose not to go through the hassle of filling out the paperwork for a disability determination. He added that getting a disability diagnosis is more than just having a good doctor, for it affects how he moves through society and what jobs he has. "It is more than just do I have a good provider or can I find a good provider. Is the system working for me in a way that I can survive in society? For a lot of people, that answer is no, unfortunately," said Link.

Thornton recalled how she had waited six months to get an appointment with her doctor—a time when she was anxious and praying that the doctor would listen to her—only to have him tell her he did not want her as a patient. Frustrated at having to start over, she waited a year before she saw a different provider and had the surgery she should have had earlier.

An unidentified workshop participant asked Lagu to talk about the systemic changes that need to occur. She replied that change must start in medical school and during medical training. She also suggested that physician attitudes would change quickly if they could bill at a higher level for working with patients with a disability and that hospitals would change their behavior quickly if accommodating people with disabilities was included in their accreditation process. Lagu said she has gotten pushback on this idea because it would treat a person with a disability differently. Chin agreed with Lagu that there must be structural reforms, such as designing clinics to be accessible and establishing longer appointment times for conducting disability evaluations.

Link said there is a fundamental tension between the medical model of disability that looks to cure or eradicate impairments versus a rights-based model of disability that acknowledges it is okay to be disabled and provides the right accommodations and access for people with a disability to thrive. "As long as our rights-based model is based on the medical model of disability, you are going to have problems with disabled people trying to access any type of social equality in that framework," said Link. "I do not know how to fix that, but that is something that we have to admit before we can do any real work."

Vincent Nibali asked the panelists for their thoughts on how to extract knowledge about community care and support—information that will not be in an EHR—for SSA's use. Thornton commented that researchers should think about how to access community knowledge and include that in a disability determination. For example, centers for independent living could produce documents that would fill gaps and support a disability determination. Link added that going into communities where there is a level of distrust and asking them to disclose their disabilities is challenging. "It is going to require a lot of work to build trust before we can even get to the point of saying which members of your community are disabled or display these signs of disability," said Link. Chin said community involvement is critical for many equity issues and raises the question of what participation means. There is a difference, for example, between a community advisory group and a group involved consistently in decision making.

Thornton pointed to the need to develop a specific definition of disability. In her case, after she had a spinal fusion, her employer sent her a letter informing her she was not disabled enough to qualify for disability, and two weeks later she received another letter saying she was too disabled to return to work and was being severed from the company. "This company is using multiple different definitions and understanding of disability to detrimentally affect my life without speaking [to me] and understanding what is going on."

Kenrick Cato, Professor of Informatics, University of Pennsylvania, asked the panelists for examples of cultural change that improved this situation. Link said that the process must start with education and getting people to understand that increasing accessibility for disabled people increases access for everyone. Thornton commented that filling out a form at a first visit to a provider and checking a race box is often where a practice's understanding of who one is as a person stops. However, her cultural understanding would differ from Lagu's cultural understanding, so these differences will cause significant issues. Chin added that the only way to change cultural attitudes is to have in-person experiences with individuals of different cultural backgrounds. "In the case of a person with disabilities, it cannot just be statistics and quantitative data. It cannot just be abstract stories. It has to be in person and [include] sharing of lived experience and honest discussions. That really is our only chance," said Chin.

Lagu said she has great hope for the medical profession because there is a grassroots movement among medical students and faculty to incorporate disability education into the medical curriculum and clinical training. "We have seen buy-in from our health system and a real willingness to change attitudes and structural barriers," said Lagu.

5

Health Disparities and the Disability Application Process

Key Messages from Individual Speakers

- Ableism and inaccessibility are the root causes of health inequities for people with disabilities, and addressing those inequities requires tackling both root causes simultaneously. (Swenor)
- Disability data is a key component for changing the paradigm on health equity for people with disabilities, but there are not enough good data that reflect the disability community in the ways it wants to be reflected. (Swenor)
- Supplemental Security Income benefits fall below the federal poverty level of $15,000 a year. (Perret)
- The disability determination process does not account for the effect of life experiences, consider homelessness to be an indicator of functional impairment, or understand the effects of childhood trauma and its link to substance use. (Perret)

The workshop's fourth session focused on the intersection of health disparities and the disability application process, including challenges in negotiating the Social Security Administration's (SSA's) disability application process, obtaining objective medical evidence, and providing SSA with medical and other records or attending a consultative examination. The three speakers in the session were Bonnielin Swenor, the endowed professor of disability health and justice at Johns Hopkins School of Nursing and founder and director of the Johns Hopkins Disability Health Research Center; D'Sena' Warren, a disability advocate; and Yvonne M. Perret, executive director of the Advocacy and Training Center in Cumberland, Maryland. Following the three presentations, Amanda Alise Price, planning committee member and chief scientific diversity officer and the director of the Office of Health Equity at the *Eunice Kennedy Shriver* National Institute of Child Health and Human Development, moderated a question-and-answer session with the panelists.

USING DATA TO ADVANCE HEALTH EQUITY FOR PEOPLE WITH DISABILITIES

Bonnielin Swenor said people with disabilities face many health inequities that are largely unaddressed (Figure 5-1) (Krahn et al., 2015). In addition to health inequities, people with disabilities face inequities in the social determinants of health (Figure 5-2), with intersectionalities between race, ethnicity, and disability (Figure 5-3) (Varadaraj et al., 2021). For example, people with

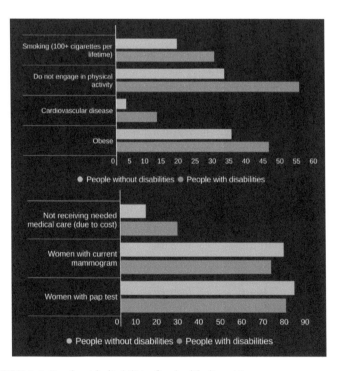

FIGURE 5-1 People with disabilities face health disparities.
SOURCES: Swenor presentation, April 4, 2024. Data from Krahn et al., 2015.

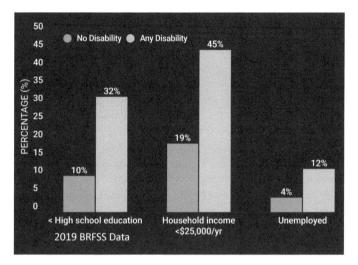

FIGURE 5-2 Disability inequities.
NOTE: BRFSS = Behavioral Risk Factors Surveillance System.
SOURCES: Swenor presentation, April 4, 2024. Data from Varadaraj et al., 2021.
JAMA Network Open. CC-BY-NC-ND.

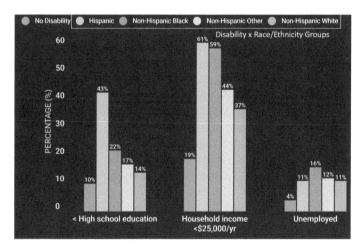

FIGURE 5-3 Intersectional disability inequities.
SOURCES: Swenor presentation, April 4, 2024. Data from Varadaraj et al., 2021.
JAMA Network Open. CC-BY-NC-ND.

disabilities who are Hispanic and Black face the highest percentage of inequities across the social determinants of health.

Ableism and inaccessibility are the root causes of health inequities for people with disabilities, and addressing those inequities requires tackling both root causes simultaneously, said Swenor. Ableism, she said, is a true threat to health equity for everyone in society. One definition of ableism says that ableism is rooted in the assumption that nondisabled people are the ideal (Morris and Alcantara, 2023). "That is what we are taught by society, in schools of public health, schools of medicine, and schools of nursing," said Swenor. "We need to challenge that idea." One study found, for example, that 82 percent of physicians believe that people with significant disabilities have worse quality of life than nondisabled people, and only 40 percent of physicians are confident about their ability to provide the same quality of care to patients with disabilities, a figure Swenor found concerning given that people with disabilities are the largest minoritized group in the United States. In addition, only 56.5 percent of physicians strongly agreed that they welcomed patients with a disability into their practice, which is discriminatory, said Swenor (Iezzoni et al., 2021).

Aside from ableism as a driver of health inequities, ableism also creates challenges with accessibility that act as barriers to information, interactions, services, programs, facilities, and environments, said Swenor. Access, she added, must be equivalent to ease of use. For her, with a visual disability, tasks can take five times as long to complete as someone without a disability, and that is not true access. "The goal post should not be 'Can I do it, yes or no.' We have to think about what is often called the disability tax, the extra time it must take me to do the thing I am trying to do," she said.

Swenor referred to Tara Lagu's comment that some doctors admit they do not want patients with disabilities and added that some office doctors whose office scales could not accommodate wheelchairs told their patients to go to a supermarket, grain elevator, cattle processing plant, or zoo to be weighed. "This is an example of both a lack of accessibility and ableism," said Swenor.

Disability data, she said, is a key component for changing the paradigm on health equity for people with disabilities, but there are not enough good data that reflect the disability community in the ways it wants to be reflected. Who counts depends on who is counted, she said, and unlike race, ethnicity, gender, and age, disability data are not collected routinely as part of demographic information (Reed et al., 2020). "We need to work with communities on how to improve the ways in which we collect disability data, but we must collect it," said Swenor. "Without the data, we have no opportunities to address and identify the inequities we are facing."

However, a proposed change to how the Census Bureau would collect disability data in the American Community Survey could undercount the number of disabled Americans by 20 million people. This proposed change, said Swenor, was made without engaging the disability community, and it underscores the mistaken idea that disability is a health outcome and not a demographic. It also highlights the problem of not having a precise definition of disability, which Gloria Thornton noted earlier in her remarks. Without a precise definition, it is difficult to collect data in a standardized manner and enable looking across datasets.

Regarding what health equity has to do with the disability determination process, Swenor said health equity is influenced by the interconnections between individual factors, communities and relationships, systems of power, and accessibility (Peterson et al., 2021). Individual factors include educational opportunity and the disability tax and how they affect the disability determination process. Relationship factors include provider bias, and systems of power include medical records requirements and inequities in disability data. Inaccessible forms and transit barriers are accessibility factors.

A PATIENT'S STORY

D'Sena' Warren grew up having episodic migraines from the time she was in primary school and into college, which is when she had her two boys who are now ages 14 and 10. While in college, she had a devastating car accident and incurred a traumatic brain injury that caused her to go from having 10 or fewer migraine attacks per month to 1 every day. The first neurologist she saw in 2010 told her the migraines would go away and she should take an over-the-counter medication once she started experiencing an attack. Though she recovered from the accident and graduated college, she lost her job because she was deemed too big of a risk.

In 2013, Warren began having seizures while she was pregnant with her youngest son, and the intensity of the head pain increased. Her neurologist told her this was typical with migraine patients and having a migraine daily was all in her head. One of her neurologists even commented in Warren's EHR that her mother was angry because the neurologist could not help her daughter. Warren's mother was not angry; she was advocating for her. However, the neurologist saw her as an angry Black woman. Warren, as for many chronic migraine sufferers, was told to drink more water or exercise more.

In 2018, Warren decided to apply for disability because of the daily seizures she was experiencing on top of the migraine attacks. When she first applied, she did it herself. As someone with a bachelor's degree and a master's degree in rehabilitation science, she felt capable of doing so, but some words on the forms were unintelligible to her. She also only included her seizure condition, believing that was the most relevant disability. After being denied, she decided to apply again, only this time she sought help from a friend in medical school to help her with the language difficulties.

Once approved, Warren grew concerned that she would only receive disability payments if she had less than $2,000 in her accounts. As a single mother of two, that was a severe financial constraint, and when she finally decided to return to work with her service dog, she feared losing her benefits if she worked too much and that she would have to go through the application process again if working full-time turned out to be unfeasible.

What helped Warren the most was finding doctors who believed in her and advocated for her, and she found peace of mind by returning to work in 2020 and being around people. "It is very isolating when you are a disabled individual," she said. She started a support group during the COVID-19 pandemic, which she still attends, and she found her community online by creating an Instagram account for her service dog. Today, she enjoys advocating for the Black, Indigenous, and People of Color communities and attending Headache on the Hill, as well as being a speaker for the U.S. Pain Foundation during the pandemic.

PEOPLE WHO ARE UNHOUSED WITH
DIAGNOSES OF MENTAL ILLNESS

Yvonne M. Perret explained that the program she helped start in Baltimore to serve people who are unhoused and have mental health problems has had a 96 percent approval rate for initial applications for disability determination. This success stems from the outreach and intensive engagement with unhoused individuals that includes conducting clinical evaluations on the street. Perret said she collects and reviews medical records so she can identify gaps that need additional information, after which she writes a comprehensive, historical medical and functional report. Although she is a licensed clinical social worker whose license allows her to diagnose physical and mental health issues, SSA does not recognize her as a clinician, so she must have her reports cosigned by a physician, nurse practitioner, or physician assistant. Perret agreed with Warren that SSA's disability application needs to be translated into regular language.

The rural area where Perret lives has limited public transportation, and the nearest provider is 26 miles away. The next county over to hers has no public transportation or cab service, and there is one SSA office serving both counties. "The geography affects the entire ability to deal with the disability determination process," said Perret.

The people she serves who are unhoused and have a mental health diagnosis are desperately poor, said Perret, and their education is often substandard. Recently, for example, she served a 19-year-old with autism, depression, and other undiagnosed conditions who grew up in an abusive home. He graduated from a technical school, where he learned culinary services, and the only weakness noted on his special education report was his inability to follow a recipe. The school graduated him nonetheless and let him go even though he should have been eligible for special education services until he was 21. Instead, he was homeless. Perret and her team got him Supplemental Security Income (SSI), and he is now housed, even though SSI benefits fall below the federal poverty level of $15,000 a year. "When are we going to say it is not okay to keep people with disabilities in poverty?" asked Perret.

SSA and Maryland's Disability Determination Services (DDS) communicate by mail and phone calls—they do not text or email—but the government-provided phones her patients have run out of minutes midmonth. This creates challenges because her unhoused clients have no residence at which to receive mail. None of her clients have laptops with Wi-Fi access, and many do not have the skills to use the Social Security website even if they had Internet access. "Social Security pushes technology, and I understand that, but there is a whole population of people served by this agency for whom it does not work," said Perret. "They need to talk to a human being, and they need to talk to the same human being, which does not happen [because] Social Security does not give out the phone extensions of their claim specialists."

Another issue facing her clients because of their living situation is that they have histories of being subjected to personal violence. Research, said Perret, shows that 74 to 87 percent of long-term unhoused people have experienced violence against them (Roy et al., 2014). In addition, resources in the rural area she works in are limited, with one inadequate hospital in the area. The physical and mental health providers in her area lack cultural and racial heterogeneity, so there are no cultural matches for her clients. Mental health providers are quick to discharge people, and it can take as long as four weeks to get an appointment with a clinician who can prescribe medication.

Health care providers do not account for their patients' living situation, said Perret. "We expect people to keep those appointments, fill that prescription, take those meds, and keep doing so," said Perret. "It does not matter whether you have no childcare, whether you have no transportation, or whether you have no emotional support." In her rural community, she is the only provider who does outreach, and the state's case management program requires people to come to the office for their appointments. Though homelessness looks different in rural areas compared to urban areas, Maryland's DDS provides no training about rural versus urban differences.

Perret said the disability determination process does not account for the effect of life experiences, nor does it consider homelessness to be an indicator of functional impairment. It does not understand the effects of childhood trauma and its link to substance use. "Policy in our country does not like people who use drugs and alcohol, and that plays out in this process," said Perret. "That is not Social Security's fault. That is Congress's fault." Maryland

DDS does not request an adverse childhood experience score when considering disability, and trauma is not part of the training the disability claim processors receive. The timelines for applying for a disability determination are arbitrary, and her clients who get their mail via general delivery cannot meet 10-day deadlines. In her view, these functional challenges should be considered with the same weight as medical evidence, and often they are not.

Medical records, said Perret, are not designed to meet Maryland DDS's requirements to make a disability determination because there is rarely any functional information in EHRs. EHRs are designed to understand symptoms, make a diagnosis, and prescribe treatment, but rarely do they contain information about how a broken leg, for example, affects an individual's day-to-day life and their ability to function.

The functional areas under Social Security for people with mental health problems include something called "adapt and manage," but Perret, who has been doing her job for 30 years, has no idea what adapt and manage means. She noted the application forms include a host of yes–no questions but not enough space to describe the variability of day-to-day life for people with mental illness.

Perret said she is grateful to have the opportunity to discuss this subject, and that for many people, Social Security benefits are the only game in town, since many states no longer have public assistance programs for people with disabilities. In Maryland, one of the wealthiest states, public assistance for individuals with disabilities is about $300 a month. Moreover, many communities treat unhoused people as criminals, which appalls her.

The suggestions Perret offered to improve this situation included:

- Training SSA and DDS staff on homelessness, trauma, poverty, cognitive impairments from trauma, and mental illness.
- Establishing time frames that account for one's living situation.
- Implementing a culture of service instead of one focusing on fraud.
- For new staff, ensuring that an experienced staff person reviews all decisions by new staff members.
- For SSA and DDS, adding text and email to the list of communication modes they use.
- For SSA and DDS, partnering with community providers who serve this population.
- Having consultative examination providers note the time they begin and end their sessions as part of their reports.
- Using treating sources for consultative examinations and giving extra weight to their information.
- Ensuring that DDS considers drug and alcohol use per requirements and reviews every claim at the DDS that includes those allegations.

Currently, someone with a substance or alcohol use disorder is denied disability coverage.

Perret said the desperation of claimants is profound, with SSA benefits being the only lifeline for many. People's experiences and their effects are ongoing and require understanding in determining disability. "It is beyond time for us to say in policy and practice that not having a home in the United States is unacceptable and that having housing is a right," said Perret. Funding an array of mental health services in every community is necessary and must happen, especially for children. She noted that the disregard about the lack of affordable housing is at a crisis level, and said service, not judgment, must be the culture of SSA and DDS.

Q&A WITH THE PANELISTS

Amanda Alise Price opened the discussion by asking Swenor how disability health inequities could be better considered in the disability determination process. Swenor replied that these inequities are baked into every step of the process yet are profoundly underaddressed and underacknowledged. Revising the disability process will require working closely with the disability community and even putting people from the community in charge of changing the process. She commented that these inequities exist because the system views people claiming to have a disability as frauds and fakers. "That is the basis of the process," said Swenor.

Vincent Nibali noted that SSA's definition of disability is based on a person's ability to work, and he asked the panelists for their advice on how to collect information on other aspects that affect a person, such as homelessness, being a single parent, or living in a rural area, and account for that information in the disability determination process. "We do not want to add more steps, but how do we get that information if we do not put out another form?" Nibali asked.

Perret replied that homelessness is indicative of functional difficulty, and being homeless is flagged by the field office to give a claim priority at DDS. Including a simple question such as "Do you have a place to live?" or "How long have you not had a place to live?" would provide that information. The Directory of Occupational Titles also needs to be updated to reflect local and regional economies. "My folks cannot move from Maryland to Alaska to be fishermen," said Perret. She also recommended that SSA should use text messaging and stop standing out as a monolith and instead be part of the community. She also called for SSA's internal culture to become one of service. Swenor added that she recognizes that as a benefit program, there are decisions to be made, but having to prove without a shadow of a doubt someone is meeting some threshold of disability is antiquated and a burden.

Joy Amaryllis Johnson remarked that many people she works with try to apply for disability on their own or with a social worker, but the minute they get an attorney that does Social Security benefits, they get approved. What this leads to is distrust in the system and the belief that the process is rigged to favor lawyers. Perret added that people get approved at hearings because it is the first time the person making a determination gets to see the individual.

Joanne Oport, from Africans for Mental Health, said it is frustrating to know that individuals living with mental illness who seek Social Security disability benefits must get legal assistance after receiving a denial. She also noted that the policies and eligibility criteria are not realistic considering the lived experiences of those with a mental illness that varies in severity over time.

Perret suggested training the people who make disability determinations to let the claimant know exactly what information is missing and how to fill in the gaps. Swenor noted that as a data scientist, she sees this boiling down to inequities and bias in health care records and the way they are being interpreted. Lagu added that doctors also need training to understand SSA language and how to help their patients provide the required information. To her, it is shameful that there is a sub-industry of lawyers making huge amounts of money off the process, to which Perret responded that what people need help with is filling in clinical gaps, which requires help from a doctor, not a lawyer. Warren suggested that SSA establish a 24-hour call line to assist claimants, particularly with wording or verbiage that is unclear.

6

Mitigating the Effect of
Health Disparities in the
SSA Disability Determination Process

Key Messages from Individual Speakers

- There cannot be a good disability determination process without considering equity. It is dangerous, in some ways, to marginalize equity issues as something separate as opposed to being integral to everything the Social Security Administration does in the disability determination process. (Chin)
- There are people who have lived experience with disability who also have lived experience designing, developing, and using electronic health records (EHRs). Perhaps those individuals should be involved in efforts to improve the ability of EHRs to capture more useful information on disability. (Petersen)

In the final session of the first day of the workshop, Michael V. Stanton, planning committee member, licensed clinical health psychologist, and associate professor of public health at California State University, East Bay, moderated a discussion among some of the speakers from previous panel sessions. The goal was to brainstorm possible approaches to mitigate the effects of the health inequities discussed in those earlier sessions on the disability determination process. The panelists for this session were Marshall H. Chin, Bonnielin Swenor, Monika Mitra, D'Sena' Warren, and Yvonne M. Perret.

Stanton opened the discussion by asking if there is anything that can be done to simultaneously address disability and health inequities, and improve the disability designation process. One step the Social Security Administration (SSA) should take, said Mitra, is to hire people who have lived experience with disability and who have worked to support people with disabilities. She also suggested improving data systems to better understand intersectionalities and the interconnectedness of the social determinants of health and disability. In addition to better data, Perret suggested increasing research to generate practice-based evidence.

Perret also thought forming a work collaborative comprising members representing different aspects of the social determinants, such as transportation and housing, health practitioners, and individuals with lived experience, could develop ideas that would improve outcomes and provide better support for people with disabilities without bringing about a massive shift in these systems. Such a collaborative could lead to efforts that operate outside of the current silos that have created the current disjointed system that causes difficulties for people living with disabilities.

Chin remarked that there cannot be a good disability determination process without equity and that it is dangerous, in some ways, to marginalize equity issues as something separate as opposed to being integral to everything SSA does in the disability determination process. Having said that, he offered three points regarding solutions. First, the goal of the determination process should not be to minimize fraud but to provide a fair and just opportunity for people with disabilities to enjoy good health. Taking that perspective would enable identifying the key checkpoints in the process and determine, for example, if the data or standards for defining disability are biased and if the process reflects the perspectives of those who have lived experience with disability. Second, there are no shortcuts to achieving equity. There are technical issues to address—are the data biased, for example—and culture change that needs to occur so that advocacy and health care organizations and SSA buy into the idea of a fair and just opportunity for health. At the same time, the business case must align with culture change.

Swenor commented that pursuing health equity is a never-ending journey. SSA is part of that journey and needs to be accountable, but there also should be accountability structures for the many communities that serve people with disabilities. She said there needs to be a growth mindset that accepts that things will not be perfect all the time, and the important point is to keep working to improve the system and to remember that people with lived experience are the real experts who need to be involved when improving the system. Mitra added that the end goal is not that SSA is providing benefits to those who need them. The end goal is to improve the quality of life and well-being of people with disabilities.

HELPING CLINICIANS HELP THEIR PATIENTS

Stanton asked the panelists for their ideas on how to guide clinicians to work within the system to move along that journey to health equity. One thing to do, replied Perret, is to tell clinicians, particularly prescribing clinicians, that by providing information, they are not deciding disability. "Part of the reluctance of the medical providers to provide information is they say 'I do not want to be the one saying whether or not [the person is disabled],'" she explained, adding that medical training should send the message that providing this information is part of health care, not outside of it. Mitra added that it is crucial for medical education to include disability training and how social determinants interact with disability to affect their patients' health.

Chin noted that clinicians are just one part of a larger ecosystem that includes SSA, providers, the health care system, community advocates, and others. Siloing the problem—just training clinicians, for example—will not solve the problem if the clinicians are working in a system that does not give them time to do a good assessment of a patient. He suggested taking an implementation science view of looking at the problem as a whole, not as individual, unconnected pieces. Perret said politicians are also part of the ecosystem, because if they are not on board with funding Social Security benefits for people with disabilities and solid clinical assessments, the focus will continue to be on withholding benefits and withholding care.

Warren commented that clinicians need to understand that every person with a disability experiences pain differently and that many people are good at masking their pain. She also called for increasing disability payments and the limit on savings that a person can have to receive financial support, an idea Perret said she supports.

ISSUES WITH THE EHR

Warren also noted that some clinicians gaslight their patients and color the electronic health records (EHRs) in a way that minimizes how a disability affects the individual. Perret added that when making a disability determination, everything the claimant says is an allegation and not evidence, as opposed to what is in the individual's medical record. For example, if a person with a disability tells their doctor they are in pain, but they are smiling and moving well, the doctor may record what they see as opposed to what the patient reports. Addressing this type of bias that tarnishes a medical record is challenging, said Amanda Price.

Perret said a problem she has seen with EHRs that is detrimental for people with mental health challenges is they now have a checklist of symptoms without elaboration, which does not do justice to an individual's experience. Stanton agreed, adding that research shows that the same symptoms in two patient populations of different ethnicities will get different diagnoses (Coleman et al., 2016; Schwartz and Blankenship, 2014; Vanderminden and Esala, 2018). "There definitely is an element of subjectivity on the provider end that probably colors the medical record," said Stanton.

Amy J. Houtrow then asked if the specialists who perform consultative examinations on behalf of people going through the disability determination process are biased in ways similar to other health professions. Chin said the weakness of the current system is that it relies on a review that it is subjective and not transparent. More delineated definitions of the criteria used in these reviews would make the process more transparent. Another approach would be to have a panel of medical experts and people with lived experience making these determinations.

Carolyn Petersen, from the Mayo Clinic, pointed out that there are people who have lived experience with disability who also have lived experience designing, developing, and using EHRs. Perhaps those individuals should be involved in efforts to improve the ability of EHRs to capture more useful information on disability.

INCORPORATING PATIENT VOICES IN RESEARCH

Jonathan Platt asked the panelists how they incorporate patient voices in their research. First, replied Swenor, include researchers with disabilities. Second, partner with people in the community at all stages of a project and provide meaningful compensation. She said that many of her colleagues subscribe to the idea that the experts are the people with diverse perspectives in the disability community. She disagreed vehemently with the view among some researchers that including people with lived experience makes research less vigorous. Petersen did as well, adding,

> When we say that a person with a disability and their work are less legitimate because of that disability, we are normalizing a certain other type of experience that trends White, trends male, trends certain gender and sex and sexual experience, and excludes older people, and has an array of other characteristics attached to it. In fact, a person who has a disability and has trained in a research process program brings additional insight that can be applied in the same way that others who have personal characteristics bring perspectives that help them to better develop research questions and expand the field.

Chin said he and his colleagues include full-blown, community-based participatory research in their work. He added that having at least three people with lived experience on an advisory committee leads to better work on improving health equity. "It is clear that the lived experience of persons with disabilities is underutilized," he said.

Mitra commented that she leads a research center where 50 percent of the team members have disabilities. Her center also involves people with lived experience as researchers on studies funded by the National Institutes of Health (NIH). The last two NIH requests for applications focused on disability and included the need to include the voices of people with lived experience. However, the grants resulting from those requests do not allow compensating those individuals for any accommodations they need to make to participate in the project.

7

The Health Record in Depth

Key Messages from Individual Speakers

- With electronic health record–based (EHR) tools, good, complete, and expressive notes and structured data can improve care quality and efficiency. (Rosenbloom)
- The digital divide leads to interventions that are not effective or that do not reach all populations equally, further exacerbating health inequities. (Del Fiol)
- Policy is an important driver of data collection. Mandating that health systems capture social determinants of health will drive a high level of data completeness in the appropriate fields in the EHR. (Adler-Milstein)
- Machine learning models, and specifically deep neural network models trained using annotated text, can identify social determinants of health from free text in EHRs. (Vydiswaran)
- The gold standard for information about an individual is what the individual says about themselves. (Adler-Milstein, Kawamoto)

The second day of the workshop opened with a panel exploring issues regarding how the electronic health record (EHR) affects disability determinations. The four speakers for this panel were S. Trent Rosenbloom, vice chair for faculty affairs and professor of biomedical informatics at Vanderbilt University Medical Center and director of the MyHealth at Vanderbilt patient portal, who discussed the basics of EHR documentation; Guilherme Del Fiol, professor and vice chair for research in the University of Utah's Department of Biomedical Informatics, who discussed the challenge of bias in EHRs and clinical documentation; Julia Adler-Milstein, professor of medicine, chief of the division of clinical informatics and digital transformation, and director of the Center for Clinical Informatics and Improvement Research at the University of California, San Francisco, who discussed how technology can pull information about social determinants of health from the EHR; and V. G. Vinod Vydiswaran, associate professor of learning health sciences at the University of Michigan Medical School and associate professor of information in the University of Michigan's School of Information, who spoke about using narrative expressive documentation. Following the four presentations, Kensaku Kawamoto, planning committee member, professor of biomedical informatics and the associate chief medical information officer at the University of Utah, and founding director of ReImagine EHR, moderated a discussion among the panelists.

CURRENT STATE OF CLINICAL DOCUMENTATION IN THE EHR

S. Trent Rosenbloom discussed the basics of how providers produce clinical notes and why. The goal of clinical documentation, he said, is to create a record of observations, impressions, plans, and activities from clinical care, usually tied to specific, billable encounters between patients and their caregivers and clinicians or health care organizations. Clinical documentation can include narrative notes using a standard, structured format about what happened at an encounter and data points, such as laboratory test results. Using computers for clinical documentation dates back to the earliest computers based on punch cards, he added.

The most common way to document an encounter in the EHR uses templates, which are structured forms with space for the clinician to enter information. Templates, said Rosenbloom, can create massive notes that are unreadable. He noted that most patients and their caregivers are storytellers, and the role of the clinician is to capture their patients' stories and replicate them in a clinical note in the EHR. Since documentation can be burdensome, physicians might shift the job of entering information into the EHR to a nurse, scribe, or medical student. Newer approaches to documenting an encounter include having multiple people collaboratively create a note using a wiki or other technology and having a computer record a clinician–patient encounter and using an artificial intelligence (AI) application to transcribe the recording into the EHR. Optical character recognition on handwritten clinical notes is another method for documenting an encounter in the EHR.

Rosenbloom explained that structured entry approaches make it easy to reuse information and compile information across EHRs, but they can be inefficient and inhibit capturing a complete narrative about an encounter. In contrast, entering a note directly maximizes storytelling and expressivity, but makes it difficult to reuse information.

Clinical documentation, said Rosenbloom, takes time away from interacting with patients, and often, clinicians spend time after work entering information into the EHR. Creating documentation is a burden and is an increasingly recognized contributor to clinician burnout, medical errors, hospital-acquired infections, and decreased clinician and patient satisfaction. Burden, he said, is an imbalance between what a clinician likes to do and what they have to do to get paid and ensure there is a legal record of the care provided. One issue is there is no clear standard for high-quality clinical documentation, and another is that a lack of integration into the workflow can increase documentation burden.

Regarding burden, research has found that outpatient physicians spend 16 minutes per patient interacting with the EHR, with 11 percent of that time spent after hours and on weekends. Nurses, said Rosenbloom, now spend 19 to 35 percent of their shift on documentation, up from 9 percent when medical records were kept on paper, and hospital nurses document an average of one data point every 49 to 88 seconds. While the burden is real, he noted that not all documentation is a burden. With EHR-based tools, good, complete, and expressive notes and structured data can improve care quality and efficiency, he said.

BIASES IN EHR DOCUMENTATION AND ITS EFFECT ON CLINICAL CARE

Guilherme Del Fiol said the widespread adoption of EHR systems is powering data-driven interventions to improve health care delivery, both in terms of clinical decision support and patient engagement. Clinical decision support systems are EHR tools that try to help health care professionals make better decisions and carry out those decisions more efficiently. Patient engagement tools include patient portals, along with emails and text messages that health care systems and providers send. Del Fiol said a substantial body of evidence shows that these tools help improve health care delivery (Bright et al., 2012; Chen et al., 2023; Han et al., 2019), but there is also evidence of a digital divide, at both the clinic and patient levels (Kan et al., 2024; Saeed and Masters, 2021). The digital divide leads to interventions that are not effective or that do not reach all populations equally, further exacerbating health inequities (Boyd et al., 2023a,b).

There has been near-universal adoption of EHRs, largely the result of the Affordable Care Act's Meaningful Use incentives. However, said Del Fiol, while even low-resource settings are using EHRs, they are less likely to adopt advanced clinical decision support tools and patient engagement functions (Adler-Milstein et al., 2017; Kruse et al., 2016). Low-resource settings also lack the capacity to optimize clinical decision support tools and to establish governance over their use, both critical for optimal functioning and effectiveness (Kawamanto et al., 2018; Wright et al., 2011). These clinics can adopt these tools and use them effectively with technical assistance, such as the assistance provided by the Centers for Disease Control and Prevention's Colorectal Cancer Prevention Program.[1] Under the auspices of this program, Del Fiol's team is working with 13 low-resource, rural federally qualified health centers (FQHCs) in Utah to help them fine-tune their EHRs so they provide reminders to clinicians that patients are due for colorectal cancer screenings and implement text messaging–based patient reminders. As a result, colorectal cancer screening rates at these FQHCs doubled after implementing these tools.

Del Fiol noted the concept of data poverty and provided a definition:

> The inability for individuals, groups, and populations to benefit from digital health advances due to health data disparities, which can perpetuate or amplify existing and known health care disparities affecting marginalized and historically underserved populations. (Ibrahim et al., 2021)

The basic idea is that people who do not have data in an EHR or are underrepresented in the EHR will not benefit from data-driven interventions, which can amplify inequities. The result is two types of bias—representativeness and information presence—with significant downstream effects. Representative bias refers to there being groups disproportionately represented in EHRs, largely because they do not have access to care, so their data will not be in EHRs. For groups that have access to care, there may still be disproportionately less complete or accurate data in EHRs.

As an example, the Broadening the Reach, Impact, and Delivery of Genetic Services (BRIDGE) trial was designed to use family history to tailor prevention strategies for a variety of conditions, including cancer, where 13 percent of the U.S. population is at elevated risk of hereditary cancer (Scheuner et al., 2010). Since most people and providers do not know this, almost everyone who would benefit do not get tested for cancer. The BRIDGE trial, said Del Fiol, used a population-based algorithm to identify eligible patients. He and his collaborators scanned EHRs according to certain rule-based criteria to find eligible people who could benefit from genetic testing and notify them proactively via an automated chatbot, written by health com-

---

[1] Available at https://www.cdc.gov/cancer/crccp/index.htm (accessed April 5, 2024).

munication experts, to provide educational information about genetic testing and offering them access to genetic testing by clicking "Yes, I would like to get tested." Those who clicked *Yes* then received a saliva-collection kit at their home, which they would mail to the laboratory and receive the results.

Del Fiol and his collaborators scanned records for nearly 446,000 individuals seen at the University of Utah and New York University, identifying over 22,000 individuals, or 5 percent of the population screened, who would benefit from direct testing (Kaphingst et al., 2021). The research team recruited approximately 3,000 of these individuals and randomized them to receive standard genetic counseling or receive information from the chatbot. Some 15 percent of the people completed genetic testing, but a secondary analysis of the data found important disparities in family history documentation, or information presence bias (Bradshaw et al., 2024; Chavez-Yenter et al., 2022). "Historically marginalized groups in the trial were about half as likely to have family history documentation, and therefore, they could not meet the algorithm criteria," said Del Fiol. "If they did not meet the algorithm criteria, they were not included in the trial and could not benefit from genetic testing."

The secondary analysis also found representativeness bias. Even for individuals who met the algorithm criteria, those in marginalized groups were less likely to have a patient portal account. "No portal account, you cannot communicate with the health system and you are not in the trial," said Del Fiol. Even those individuals from marginalized communities who had patient portal accounts were less likely to access their messages, and even if they answered their messages, they were less likely to use the chatbot. "It requires some digital literacy and, at the end, the downstream effect, they do not have the benefit of genetic testing," he explained.

Digital exclusion, said Del Fiol, is a "super" social determinant of health (Sieck et al., 2021), given that people need digital technology to access health care, find resources in the community, buy food, get transportation, and obtain an education (Figure 7-1). "Being excluded from the digital environment contributes to health disparities," he said.

To reduce inequities, Del Fiol said it is important to think carefully about the design of digital interventions so they increase inclusion rather than exclusion. One step would be to ask patients when they come to the clinic if they have access to digital technology and the patient portal. For those who do not, digital navigators—with training, community health workers could serve this role—could help those individuals. Another idea would be to have proactive patient outreach and connection with services via patient portals, text messaging, and chatbots for those who are connected digitally. Today, 97 percent of people in the United States have access to phones with text-messaging capability.

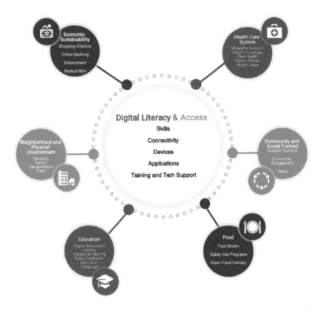

FIGURE 7-1 Digital inclusion plays a role in many social determinants of health.
SOURCES: Del Fiol presentation, April 5, 2024; Sieck et al., 2021. https://doi.org/10.1038/s41746-021-00413-8. CC BY 4.0.

CAPTURING SOCIAL DETERMINANTS WITH
HEALTH INFORMATION TECHNOLOGY

Julia Adler-Milstein said EHRs have become somewhat of a Frankenstein tool, where they have been adapted to serve different purposes for different contexts. It is hard to say confidently that every EHR will have a particular type of data.

In 2014, the Institute of Medicine released two reports that pushed the need for EHRs to capture social and behavioral determinants given how important those are to understanding an individual's health and identifying optimal treatments (Institute of Medicine, 2014a,b).[2] In 2016, the 21st Century Cures Act contained a set of policies that pushed for those data to be readily exported and shared from EHRs via interoperability and data standards. The U.S. Core

---

[2] As of March 2016, the Health and Medicine Division of the National Academies of Sciences, Engineering, and Medicine continues the consensus studies and convening activities previously carried out by the Institute of Medicine (IOM). The IOM name is used to refer to reports issued prior to July 2015.

Data Set for Interoperability is the standardized set of health data classes and constituent data elements for nationwide, interoperable health information exchange. While this is the standard, the problem is that the data that are actually available depends on what local health systems are capturing.

A 2019 national survey of ambulatory physicians found that 76 percent were aware their EHR could record social determinants of health data, while 12 percent did not think their EHR could do that and another 12 percent were unsure (Iott et al., 2022). A subsequent 2022 survey found that 81 percent of the physicians were documenting social determinants in their clinical notes in free text form, 61 percent were also documenting social determinants in some structured data field, which could be either a checkbox or a button, and 46 percent said they were using diagnostic codes for social determinants of health (Iott et al., 2023). For family medicine physicians, 61 percent said they documented social determinants in their clinical notes, while 52 percent also documented them via structured data fields.

Adler-Milstein and her collaborators collected similar data from hospitals, finding that 83 percent were collecting data on patient health-related social needs and 54 percent were doing so routinely (Chang and Richwine, 2023). What this means is the data would be available, but in a variety of places in the EHRs.

When Adler-Milstein and her colleagues did a deep dive into their own institution's EHR, they found that inpatient nursing questions contained the most data on social determinants of health (Iott et al., 2024), largely because California passed a regulation that nurses had to document a person's housing status for every admission. "One key takeaway is that policy is an important driver. If you are mandated to capture social determinants of health data, you will probably see high completeness of data in that field," said Adler-Milstein.

About half of the patient EHRs examined had social history text, and about half had social determinants data in social work notes. To determine the accuracy and completeness of these data and the extent to which the documentation represents the true prevalence of social risk, Adler-Milstein and her colleagues surveyed patients and asked them directly about their social determinants of health and compared that to what they found in EHR data (Figure 7-2). The results showed there was a vast gap between the level of social determinants and needs that patients reported and what was in the EHR.

Efforts to use geocoding and various measures such as the Social Vulnerability Index, Area Deprivation Index, and neighborhood stress score as proxies for social determinants that could supplement the EHR from a patient's zip code found important limitations. One study of over 35,000 patients from a large network of safety net clinics found that almost 30 percent of their populations screened positive for one or more social risks, but 42 percent of the patients with at least one social risk lived in a neighborhood that was

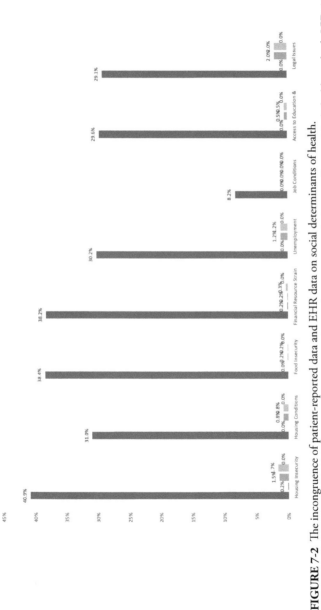

FIGURE 7-2 The incongruence of patient-reported data and EHR data on social determinants of health.
NOTES: Dark blue = survey report needed; gray = clinical note documentation during enrollment visit; light blue = both ICD-10 Z Code and note documentation during enrollment visit; red = ICD-10 Z Code documentation during enrollment visit; and yellow = ICD-10 Z Code and/or Clinical Note Documentation during enrollment visit.
SOURCES: Adler-Milstein presentation, April 5, 2024; Iott et al. 2024. *Journal of the American Medical Informatics Association.* Volume 31, Issue 3, pages 714-719, by permission of Oxford University Press.

not defined as being disadvantaged (Cottrell et al., 2020). Another study of a Medicare Advantage population found the agreement between area-level and individual-level social risk ranged from 53 percent to 77 percent (Brown et al., 2023). "It is probably better to use these proxies, but it is definitely not going to solve the whole problem," said Alder-Milstein.

Regarding the quality of social determinants of health data in EHRs, she pointed to a 2022 systematic review that looked at this very issue (Cook et al., 2021). In the 76 studies reviewed, the most common issues were completeness and plausibility—are the data values believable and accurate—for individual-level data.

In summary, the data show there is high awareness that EHRs can capture social determinants data, and the reported use is high across all potential methods of documentation. However, there are many methods used to collect these data, and only about one-third of those data are documented using structured diagnostic codes. Regarding actual use of these data, the evidence is limited. At her health system, the levels of documentation were low unless mandated, in which case it was high, or via free text, in which case the level of documentation was moderate. Completeness and plausibility shortcomings reflect on the quality of the data, with the levels of social determinants documentation dramatically underrepresenting self-reported levels and area-level proxy measures, producing noisy data.

As a final comment, Adler-Milstein said there are a great deal of data available on the social determinants of health. However, while that is a good starting point, she also said,

> I do not think we can move forward confidently, especially when we are at the point of thinking about eligibility for services, to say these are going to be a robust source of data to tell us who really is or is not eligible for different types of services based on social determinants.

THE IMPORTANCE OF FREE TEXT IN EHRs AND THE ROLE OF ARTIFICIAL INTELLIGENCE

V. G. Vinod Vydiswaran explained that data in EHRs come in two forms: structured in defined fields and unstructured, which are data available in notes and radiology reports, for example. Unstructured data are not readily searchable or available for downstream decision-making tasks. He noted, too, the abundance of text data in health, whether as books and the peer-reviewed literature, paper-based medical records, or prescriptions, that may not find its way into the EHR. Medical natural language processing is an area of AI that synthesizes information from a variety of unstructured data sources to generate insights, such as whether a treatment worked or not.

Vydiswaran discussed how natural language processing can identify cohorts from the narrative data in EHRs by identifying patients who meet certain selection criteria. For example, a search of text data in an EHR might identify men who engage in low-risk alcohol use by spotting text in notes stating that a male patient lives with his wife and drinks two glasses of wine nightly. However, if that same individual were female, they would be in a high risk of alcohol use cohort because of a different defined threshold.

AI-powered models, said Vydiswaran, can identify disease better than just using International Classification of Diseases (ICD) codes. Continuing with the example above, a search of ICD codes in EHRs identified only 29 percent of patients who were high-risk alcohol users. In contrast, natural language processing, by looking for information such as how many drinks a person has or whether they have had a driving while intoxicated citation or come into the emergency department after falling in a bar, identified 87 percent of the patients with risky alcohol behavior (Vydiswaran et al., 2024).

Vydiswaran said that machine learning models, and specifically deep neural network models trained using annotated text, can identify social determinants of health from free text in EHRs (Lybarger et al., 2023a,b). Researchers have also used deep neural network models to identify inequities in telehealth use during the COVID-19 pandemic via EHR analyses of notes providers entered after successful and failed telehealth visits (Buis et al., 2023). Patients who completed telehealth visits were more likely to be younger than 65 years old, female, White, and have no significant comorbidities or disabilities than those who only canceled or missed telehealth appointments. A subsequent analysis identified those patients who had technical difficulties with their telehealth encounter. Individuals whose primary language was Spanish, along with individuals with mobility and vision disabilities, were most likely to experience technical difficulties. Other individuals who were more likely to experience technical difficulties included those who were female, over age 65, Black or African American, or American Indian or Alaska Native, and those with hearing and cognitive disabilities.

The lesson here, said Vydiswaran, is that although EHRs are faulty, incomplete, and biased, machine learning and AI-based natural language processing can pull out information useful for downstream tasks. The positive news is that text is everywhere in health care, providing a valuable source of data that is accessible with the right tools. He reiterated that AI and deep learning methods are more effective than ICD codes alone for phenotyping patient cohorts.

Q&A WITH THE PANELISTS

After summarizing his take-home messages from the presentations, Kensaku Kawamoto commented that as Adler-Milstein noted, the gold standard for self-reported information (e.g., social determinants of health data) about an individual is what the individual says about themselves. Therefore, when applying for a Social Security disability determination, such information should come directly from the patient, not the EHR.

An unidentified workshop participant remarked that the Social Vulnerability Index as a measure of social determinants includes disability status at the county level, while the Area Deprivation Index provides information at the block level but no information about disability. They then asked if pulling data from the Social Vulnerability Index when looking at rural versus urban populations risks doing harm by pulling in data from a broader group that does not get to the needed individualized decisions. Adler-Milstein responded that it is important when trying to make a disability determination to conduct deep investigative work to understand what those sources are capturing. Given there is not a data source that provides the exact information needed in this case, the best approach is to put them together and find consistencies across the data sources that would point to populations more likely to be facing challenges based on where they live. "Our best hope is that we have enough options of different data sources that if we put them together, we can feel more confident in them," she said. The alternative, she added, is to design and validate a measure specifically fit for this purpose.

Michael V. Stanton asked the panelists to discuss how language can affect inequities. Vydiswaran answered that in his study during the COVID-19 pandemic, there was a technical issue with having three people on a telehealth visit, which were intended to be bidirectional. The solution to this problem lies in scheduling and noting in the EHR that a person has a disability or a need for a medical interpreter, for example, so when the appointment time came, that assistance would be available.

Rosenbloom said the barrier he sees with patient portal access is that they are written for people who speak English. This can create navigational challenges for individuals for whom English is not their native language, and it can make it difficult for the same individuals to access and understand educational materials available through the patient portal. Major EHR vendors have added additional language capabilities to patient portals for navigation purposes, but all information is not available in Arabic or German, for example. Beyond language issues, there are other access issues, such as the need to use one's Social Security number to access the portal. "If our patient portal requires a Social Security number to access it, you lose a lot of Spanish speakers and you lose a lot of other language speakers who do not have a U.S. Social Security number," said Rosenbloom. "If you require an email address to access it, you also lose a lot of people who do not use email and use WhatsApp."

Del Fiol agreed that language is a huge factor in EHR data. His work, for example, found that having a non-English language recorded in the EHR is the strongest predictor for not having a complete family history, or any family history, recorded in the EHR, not having access to the patient portal, and not accessing the chatbot for genetic testing. However, in a study whose goal was to increase uptake of COVID-19 testing by patients, his team used bilingual text messaging to offer to mail test kits to people's homes. The people who reviewed the grant application were skeptical that people who did not speak English would respond, but the opposite was true. People whose preferred language was Spanish had a higher response rate than those who spoke English. The key is to be intentional about making information accessible.

Elham Mahmoudi, from the University of Michigan, noted that many clinicians are not using social determinants of health information in EHRs because they do not have time. Her institution is having medical social workers look for and act on that information, though her concern is that health care systems are cutting back on their use of medical social workers. Rosenbloom agreed that time pressures play a role, but so does doctors not knowing what to do with social determinants of health information, whereas a medical social worker would.

Tara Lagu said that while asking about the social determinants of health is important, there need to be standardized questions to ask about the social determinants. Otherwise, every health system is asking different questions, making it hard to compare across systems. She has also found that the answers one gets depends on who is asking the question, making the data analysis even more challenging. Adler-Milstein added there is a tension between the call for data standards and pushback from health systems and EHR vendors about having to develop more standards. Adler-Milstein said this is a recognized problem, but she is not sure the solution will come soon.

Rupa Valdez asked the panelists if they see any changes in the data being captured and how it is being captured given that scribes are often used to record data. Rosenbloom replied that scribes are poorly studied and poorly standardized, making it difficult to generalize about what scribes are doing and translate learnings from one setting to another. Another concern with scribes is that they are a crutch that does not address the underlying problems of documentation burden and documentation quality. To him, the solution is to focus on education from the start of medical and nursing school through continuing education and having supports in practice.

Yvonne M. Perret asked if there was any research focusing on FQHCs and social determinants of health. She wants to have a tool that a community health worker could use to get information about social determinants of health and the supports needed to address them. Rosenbloom, who practices at an FQHC, said the challenge is that FQHCs have little money and cannot afford large vendor-based EHR systems, so the EHRs they have are difficult to use and cannot contribute high-quality notes or clinical documentation. These EHRs do not accommodate narrative documentation particularly well, and patients at the FQHC rarely use the patient portal. At the same time, FQHCs have certain reporting standards and therefore have methods and processes for capturing structured information.

Del Fiol said his team held focus groups with community health center clients, and the message was consistent: they are reluctant to disclose problems such as food and housing insecurity at a clinic visit. They are more likely, though, to talk to a community health worker they trust. He also noted that social determinants can change between appointments and that what is recorded in the EHR is just a snapshot of the situation at the time of an appointment. His team is trying to proactively contact patients through low-tech means such as text messaging to ask more often about social needs and to conduct a quick screening with yes-or-no questions about food and housing security, for example. A *yes* answer would prompt a community health worker to reach out to that individual.

8

The Relationship Between the
Medical Record and Health Disparities

Key Messages from Individual Speakers

- Since disability status can change over time, there needs to be consistent and regular documentation of disability status in the electronic health record (EHR). (Morris)
- There are two types of disability bias in the EHR. The first is stigmatizing language, such as *wheelchair-bound* or *retarded*, and the second is language suggesting biases and stereotypes, such as *lazy* or *noncompliant*. (Morris)
- Health care systems are having trouble implementing disability status in their EHRs. The lack of standardized tools to collect disability status in the EHR is one impediment. Another is a lack of federal, state, and local policies that require documenting disability status. (Morris)
- EHRs document health information but not the effects of impairments on individuals' lives, thereby limiting care teams' ability to recognize needs. (Petersen)
- A reliable method for documenting social drivers and disabilities is to have the patient answer directed questions through their patient-facing portal outside of the clinical setting. Sometimes, doing this in the privacy of their own homes makes it easier for patients to answer questions sensitive to them. (Laddha)

- EHRs contain data that could help identify where disability and the social determinants of health intersect. Those health care organizations that are not doing this analysis are not tracking health disparities in their organization. (Skapik)
- To realize the potential of improving care for people with disabilities, people with disabilities, their partners, and patient advocates must continue pushing for the positive uses of these data and tools and not expect it to organically occur on its own. (Petersen)

The workshop's final presentations discussed subjects such as risk indications of health disparities, differences in documentation, capturing disability status in the health record, and equity regarding medical information in the electronic health record (EHR). The four speakers were Megan Morris, associate professor of medicine at the University of Colorado Anschutz Medical Campus; Carolyn Petersen, senior editor of the www.mayoclinic.org website; Prerana Laddha, director of social care and behavioral health at Epic Systems; and Julia Skapik, medical director for informatics at the National Association of Community Health Centers. Kenrick Cato, planning committee member and professor of nursing and clinical informatics at the University of Pennsylvania and Children's Hospital of Philadelphia, moderated a question-and-answer session after the panel presentations.

DISABILITY STATUS IN EHRs

Megan Morris recounted how when she went to visit her uncle, who had a developmental disability, in the hospital after he suffered a serious fall, she found his hands tied to either side of his bed, with no access to a nurse call button. When she asked the nurse about this, the nurse told her that because he had a developmental disability, he was a danger to himself and others and did not have communication skills, so he did not need access to the call button. Morris walked the nurse back to her uncle's room and began asking him yes/no questions—including a question about a recent presidential debate; he could answer yes with a thumbs-up with his right hand and no with a thumbs-up with his left hand, and he answered correctly each time. "That team had made assumptions about David because of what was written in his medical chart, that he had a developmental disability," she said. "I believe one of the first steps to begin to address these disparities and these challenges that he experienced is through consistent documentation of disability status."

Morris explained that diagnostic codes are based on a medical model and are used to inform billing and medical treatment. A clinician documents them, and they are located throughout a patient's chart. In contrast, disability status is based on a social model, and there are two main purposes of documenting disability status in the EHR. The first is to inform the provision of accessible health care as the Americans with Disabilities Act and Affordable Care Act mandate. "If you do not know who has a disability, you cannot provide them with accommodations," said Morris. The second purpose of disability status documentation in the EHR is to identify and address disparities. Disability status needs to be self-reported, and it should appear in a prominent location in a patient's EHR. One way to elicit information about a person's disability is to ask a series of questions (Figure 8-1).

There are many reasons diagnostic codes are insufficient for identifying and addressing disparities, starting with the inconsistency with which clinicians document them. For example, a patient could have a diagnostic code related to stroke with hemiparesis in their EHR, but if the clinician at a follow-up visit does not use that code, it could mean the clinician decided not to use that code anymore, or it could be that the person has recovered from their stroke and does not have hemiparesis anymore. "Since disability status can change over time," said Morris, "we need consistent and regular documentation of disability status."

In addition, she explained, diagnostic codes do not provide information about accommodations, so if someone has a cerebral palsy diagnosis, the associated code does not say anything about that individual's specific limitations. Without knowing if the individual has difficulty with cognition, mobility, vision, or hearing, it is difficult to have necessary accommodations ready when the individual has a medical appointment.

Disability Category	Patient-Centered Disability Questionnaire
Hearing	Are you deaf, or do you have serious difficulty hearing?
Vision	Are you blind, or do you have serious difficulty seeing, even when wearing glasses?
Cognition	Do you have difficulty remembering or concentrating?
Mobility	Do you have serious difficulty walking or climbing stairs?
Activities of Daily Living (ADL)/Fine Motor	Do you have difficulty dressing or bathing?
Communication	Using your usual language, do you have difficulty communicating (for example, understanding or being understood)?
General screener	Due to a disability, do you need any additional assistance or or accommodations during your visit?

FIGURE 8-1 Disability status questions.
SOURCE: Morris presentation, April 5, 2024.

There are two types of disability bias in the EHR. The first is stigmatizing language, such as *wheelchair-bound* or *retarded*, and the second is language suggesting biases and stereotypes, such as *lazy* or *noncompliant* (Figure 8-2). Morris noted that research shows that when health care team members read biased language in the medical chart, it affects the medical care they provide and their decision making (Casau and Beach, 2022).

Morris and her colleagues have been conducting studies over the years to document disability status in the EHR. Patients, she said, support these efforts and do not object when asked about their disability status. One finding from her research points to the importance of tying disability status to the legal requirement for providing accommodations to give health care teams a reason to document this information. However, health care systems are having trouble implementing disability status in their EHRs. The lack of standardized tools to collect disability status in the EHR is one impediment. Another is a lack of federal, state, and local policies that require documenting disability status.

There are still significant biases around documenting disability status. One common statement she hears from clinicians is that documentation is great, but not for those faking a disability. Morris recalled how one director of a primary care clinic told her they could not document disability because everyone would claim low back pain and disability. "We need to think about addressing those biases and that lack of education," said Morris.

The situation is not completely dire, as there have been positive advances in the policy and research areas. For example, in July 2022, the Office of the National Coordinator for Health Information Technology released the third edition of its interoperability standards that contain elements representing disability status. In 2023, the Joint Commission released a new health equity certificate that requires disability status documentation, and in 2024, the Centers for Medicare & Medicaid Services (CMS) released the CMS

Disability Stigmatizing Language	Language that suggests biases and stereotypes
- Wheelchair- or bed-bound	Language that suggests patients are:
- Confined to a...	- Lazy
- Suffers from...	- "Faking" a disability
- Stricken with...	- Non-reliable historian
- Retarded	- Incompetent
- Handicap	- Childlike
- Special needs	- Non-compliant
- Challenged	

FIGURE 8-2 Stigmatizing language and disability bias in clinical notes.
SOURCE: Morris presentation, April 5, 2024.

Enhancing Oncology Model that requires disability status documentation. Morris noted that while the Health Resources and Services Administration requires documentation of race, ethnicity, sexual orientation, and gender identity, it does not mandate collecting disability status. "This is hampering research and advancement in this area," said Morris.

Recently, the National Institutes of Health awarded funding to Morris and colleagues to develop and evaluate workflows for consistently documenting disability status in the EHR and then use the data to inform provision of accommodations. Morris and her collaborators are working with Epic to create a standardized approach for documenting disability status. On a final note, Morris said the Disability Equity Collaborative, which includes members from health systems, providers, insurers, and patients, issued an implementation guide to help health systems integrate disability status collection into the EHR and workflow processes.

THE EHR AND WHAT IT DOES NOT TELL US

When a member of someone's care team opens their EHR, said Carolyn Petersen, they can see the individual's personal and family histories, test results, and any diagnoses. There will be treatment history, some health outcomes and patient-related outcome measures, maybe some information on social determinants of health, and perhaps some person-generated health data, such as sleep patterns and other information an individual maintains for themselves and through an agreement with their care team, though the latter is not standard. The care team can update personal and family histories; review diagnoses and previous care; check test results and patient-reported outcome measures; order tests, medications, and durable medical goods; make referrals; and schedule appointments and consultations, both internal and external.

Petersen said when people get into their EHR through their patient portal, they may see inaccurate or incomplete information, which she said can be concerning at a minimum and even enraging and frustrating. Though individuals may attempt to correct misinformation in their EHR, many EHR systems do not allow that. Regarding what gets missed in the EHR, Petersen said the EHR does not capture the effects of disability or illness on daily life. The EHR also does not capture the effects of any changes in a person's health and ability to function in all the environments and roles of which they are a part.

Petersen presented a case study involving fragrance sensitivity, an invisible disability that affects some 20 to 25 percent of people, said Petersen (de Groot, 2020). Today, over 2,000 fragrances occur in various consumer products, and a fragrance can include 10 to over 100 chemicals. Some chemicals help the fragrance linger in the air so the fragrance can persist. She said it is hard to know the chemical names of a fragrance's constituents, making them difficult to study. There are many symptoms of fragrance susceptibility, including respiratory distress, skin rashes, headaches, other neural symptoms, and sometimes nausea. Skin sensitivity tests can detect many allergens, but not all.

Regarding what the care team can do with the EHR, they can document discussions about fragrance-related issues, order tests, annotate recommendations for over-the-counter medications, prescribe medications, and create a referral to a dermatologist, allergist, or other specialists. From an individual's perspective, the patient is aware of all the challenges they encounter in trying to manage those symptoms, which can change from day to day, and they are aware of the limitations to their lives when they cannot adapt their environment or roles.

What is missing from the EHR are the reduced social interactions given the need to avoid public transportation with assigned seating because of the possibility someone wearing too much perfume will sit next to them. These things cause individuals with a sensitivity to have few career options and opportunities. They may, for example, have to work remotely or be ineligible for company-provided health care insurance, and their income may suffer, reducing their access to supportive services such as home food delivery. Finally, there are symptom-specific risks. Antihistamines, for example, may increase a person's experience with hazards; light sensitivity may make people susceptible to falls given their use of sunglasses; and nausea can increase the risk of falls that result from dizziness from skipping meals.

Petersen concluded her remarks with four key points:

1. EHRs document health information but not the effects of impairments on individuals' lives, thereby limiting care teams' ability to recognize needs.
2. People have varying degrees of health literacy and digital skills, and they may not document health and disability issues and their effect on function in the terminology of medical professionals and agencies.
3. Health conditions and disabilities are dynamic, with variable and changing effects on functions not captured in the EHR.
4. Determination of function and disability is not a function of technology but a process between an individual and their care team; technology may be a facilitator, not a solution.

SOCIAL DRIVERS OF HEALTH IN THE MEDICAL RECORD

Prerana Laddha said there is substantial focus on equitable care in the EHR resulting from its ability to collect accurate data on race, ethnicity, sexual orientation, gender identity, and social drivers. The EHR also enables compiling these data on a population level to understand where disparities in the health system are, and it can provide interventions in a provider's workflow to promote equity. She noted that over the last decade, health systems have become increasingly interested in documenting social determinants of health and addressing them for their patient population.

Laddha said her company includes validated clinical assessments to document this information in its EHR and makes the information available as a social determinants of health wheel in the patient's chart that a provider accesses in the normal course of their workflow. "Having that type of data front and center not only helps this provider make the right decision, but it is also constantly promoting equity as they are going through their patients in their busy schedule," said Laddha. There is value, too, in showing these data over time, said Laddha. For example, a clinician who sees their patient has food insecurity and connects them with Meals on Wheels can see if that connection helps the patient improve their health. She added that a reliable method for documenting social drivers and disabilities is to have the patient answer directed questions through their patient-facing portal outside of the clinical setting. Sometimes, doing this in the privacy of their own homes makes it easier for patients to answer questions sensitive to them.

Using social data promptly within workflows is something today's EHRs can do. For example, said Laddha, a scheduler can see a patient has transportation risks and contact the patient before their appointment to ask if they need a rideshare service to get them to the office. Interoperability standards, she added, can enable health systems and organizations to exchange these data so as someone moves between health systems and organizations, their data can move with them.

Laddha said EHR vendors such as her company will soon incorporate artificial intelligence (AI) tools in the EHR to extract information from clinical notes. "Clinical notes is our primary focus because we have seen statistics that over 50 percent of this social driver data still lives in clinical notes, so it is a good place for us to start extracting that information using AI," said Laddha.

Disability and accommodation needs are a part of what the EHR can capture within various workflows, including during scheduling, registration, and clinical encounters. "Just like with social drivers, having that ability to document the disability status and accommodation needs before my upcoming visit [can help] the clinic or the hospital be better prepared to accommodate me when I get there," said Laddha. She noted that she and her colleagues are working with Morris's team to standardize disability data collection to improve interoperability and visualize the information for providers.

As mentioned in an earlier presentation, providers are sometimes hesitant to document social information because they do not know how to help the individual. To address this, Laddha's company's EHR has a resource directory available. When a patient screens positive for any of the social needs in the directory, the system automatically selects some community resources and prompts the provider. She explained the automation is based on several factors, including the patient's demographics, their insurance coverage, veteran status, and location. This does not take additional time from the office visit, nor does it increase the need for documentation or to search through a list of services. The provider can text or mail these resources to the patient and communicate bidirectionally with the community providers to let them know a referral is coming.

The ability of EHRs to capture Z codes can help justify needed interventions. A patient who presents with chronic conditions exacerbated by homelessness, and whose EHR contains a Z code denoting that, can help the clinician justify the extra interventions and services the patient needs. It can also help with reimbursement, a further encouragement to document this information, said Laddha.

As she mentioned earlier, EHRs can provide information at the population level. This can enable a health system to see overall screening rates and how many people within a population are screening positive. Geographic information can also pinpoint problem areas where housing or transportation are major social drivers, enabling health systems to target those areas with strategic initiatives, such as establishing a food pantry or lobbying for an additional bus line. EHRs can help health systems analyze the effects of social drivers on health outcomes. An analysis of outcomes and social drivers might show, for example, that patients with diabetes with adverse outcomes are affected more by a lack of transportation than by an elevated A1C level.

STANDARDS AND OPPORTUNITIES

Community health centers, said Julia Skapik, arose as an outgrowth of the civil rights movement to address a lack of culturally competent health care in health care access deserts. There are five essential elements to a community health center. They are in high-need areas and provide comprehensive health and wraparound services, including enabling services or social care services. They are open to all residents regardless of insurance or the ability to pay, with a sliding scale fee based on income, and they are nonprofits governed by community boards to ensure responsiveness to local needs. Finally, they follow performance and accountability requirements regarding their administrative, clinical, and financial operations.

Today, said Skapik, the nation's 1,487 community health centers serve about 9 percent of the U.S. population, or 31.5 million people, and over 14,000 sites. They disproportionately serve underserved communities, and the majority of health center patients come from minoritized populations.

They also serve a large proportion of people who are unhoused or who are uninsured. At her health center, over 40 percent of its patients are best served in a language other than English.

Skapik, who serves as a part-time primary care physician at a community health center, commonly interacts with people with a disability. In that role, her primary goal is to help these individuals achieve and maintain their goals and functionality. However, her community health center's information technology infrastructure has a limited focus on assessing and improving functional status, understanding a patient's story, and supporting their goals. Skapik said,

> There is a duality of being a health care provider in this space because on the one hand, I genuinely want to help meet my patients' needs, and on the other hand, what I see as the activities around disability are administrative, burdensome, confusing, and frustrating.

She added that some of this frustration stems from working to document social drivers and disabilities for patients and not being reimbursed for that work.

Theoretically, the EHR has the information clinicians need, and in fact, there is many times more information in a patient's EHR than anyone will ever look at or use. What the EHR does not adequately support—and this, she said, might be a generous categorization—is functional status and disability status and the workflow around that. She also commented that medicine still treats health data as little fragments of something at one moment in time tied to a specific encounter. "We do not think about these things as episodic, so it is difficult to understand a patient's story by looking at those fragments of data," said Skapik. In her opinion, the time is right to use AI, health IT standards, and fast processing to unlock the information in the petabytes of data in an EHR.

Skapik noted that while the Office of the National Coordinator for Health Information Technology required health organizations to have access to Fast Healthcare Interoperability Resources application programming interfaces, community health centers are often last on the implementation priority list. In fact, too many community health centers do not have access to this interface. One problem with the current standards is that capturing disability status is limited to finding a Logical Observation Identifiers Names and Code that denotes an individual's disability status. What is needed, said Skapik, are sound data models built with the input of patients with lived experience and subject matter experts who understand the germane science and research.

Skapik said she dreams of the day when a dashboard tracks over time a person's functional status and sends her alerts when there are changes in an individual's functional status. This requires identifying the data providers will record over time and setting thresholds for notifying the clinician when functional status has changed. For cognitive status, there may not be an easy way to identify changes over time in the EHR. She mentioned the Pacio Project as a successful partnership that aims to create formal standards for postacute, home, and functional status improvement and build use cases before building these standards.

EHRs, said Skapik, contain data that could help identify where disability and the social determinants of health intersect. Those health care organizations that are not doing this analysis are not tracking health disparities in their organization, adding,

> If we are not setting up dashboards and support for analytics at the point of care to look at the intersection of all of these different domains, we are going to fail to see that there are some really big signals and big opportunities to address those.

Skapik mentioned the Gravity Project, which aims to accelerate the adoption of nationally recognized standards to advance identifying and acting on social determinants of health. She also briefly discussed the validated PRAPARE tool, a national standardized patient risk assessment protocol built into the EHR. PRAPARE is designed to engage patients in assessing—and importantly—addressing social determinants of health. She noted that the focus on actions to address social determinants of health is important for ameliorating the "moral hazard" people experience when asked about social determinants of health without having an intervention to deal with them. Regarding the Z codes that health care organizations use to capture social determinants of health, Skapik said they do not contain enough information to understand what a patient is experiencing.

Skapik offered suggestions for improving how the EHR can support disability. There is a concept called the care plan that aims to link these pieces of information with related information and track them over time to generate a complete picture of what is going on with a patient. The data should come from both the patient and everyone involved in the care ecosystem, including caregivers the patient authorizes to contribute data. Federal EHR regulations support this concept, she said, though one challenge is convincing the care team there is value in documenting a patient's goals and what the health care system is doing to meet those goals.

Skapik also listed opportunities to support disability in the EHR. These included:

- Standardizing disability templates and data elements;
- Enabling electronic submission of forms for disability determinations, using the model of electronic prior authorizations;

- Better supporting care teams by providing regular evaluation and documentation of a patient's functional status, cognitive and behavioral health status, social determinants of health, and health-related social needs; and
- Integrating patient-generated health data via apps and allowing them to track their own status.

Q&A WITH THE PANELISTS

Laura Jantos, from RecastHealth, asked how bidirectional communication with community services is happening and what systems community providers have that allow them to receive this information in a structured format if they do not have EHRs? Laddha replied that providing community resources has been an area her company has been working on in terms of improving the software and workflows. Her company's EHR, for example, integrates with FindHelp and Unite Us, both of which evaluate social care investments. Community-benefit organizations, said Laddha, use this software to receive electronic referrals and accept or decline them. She noted her company is working with the Gravity Project to standardize the interfaces so this software can be adopted broadly.

Maggie Downey, a former medical social worker, said she is excited about health care reforming how it addresses the social determinants of health, but she struggles with how a community resource directory, even with bidirectional communication, is better or different than a social work model, which has not meaningfully addressed the social determinants either. Laddha said what her company has seen over the last few years is that connecting patients or assessing patients for social needs is happening across different settings. Previously, she said, it was care managers, social workers, or community health workers who focused on this work, but it is now happening in hospital settings. Therefore, providing a quick and easy tool that can be automated and help workflows is what the resource directory aims to accomplish. Skapik added that developers could use the Fast Healthcare Interoperability Resources standard to create a smartphone app that social care organizations can use without needing an EHR to enter the information they want displayed and that consumers could access directly and enter information.

Amy J. Houtrow commented that if EHRs are going to document disability status and providers are biased against people with disabilities, it is surprising that patients with disabilities favor having that information in their EHR. She also noted the importance of acting on disability status and providing accommodations, yet the disability status questions Morris listed do not provide the information needed to address accommodations. Given this, she wondered how the field can get to a place that identifies what people need and provide it and not have them face discriminatory practices in health care.

Morris replied that people with disabilities have told her it is key to ask questions about disability and accommodations early, before a clinical appointment. The challenge with the questions Houtrow raised is that they must serve two purposes—identifying patients who require accommodations and tracking health inequities—that are often at odds with each other. Regarding the bias people with disabilities face, she said if someone is in a wheelchair, they will experience biases whether they are asked about their disability or not. However, acquiring that information is a first step toward providing equitable care and getting health care teams to think more explicitly about their biases.

Skapik said asking people in their own words is undervalued in health care. The advent of AI and natural language processing creates the ability to take large groups of similar disparate concepts and group them in a meaningful way, "but that is not worth anything if we do not display that information to the care team and let them understand what supports they must figure out if they are appropriately accommodating a condition," she said.

Petersen, speaking as someone who has had a disability long enough to remember when employment forms said people with physical defects need not apply, said that to realize the potential of improving care for people with disabilities, people with disabilities, their partners, and patient advocates must continue pushing for the positive uses of these data and tools and not expect it to organically occur on its own.

9

Approaches to Advancing Medical Records to Address Disparities in Disability Determinations

Key Messages from Individual Speakers

- Bias in electronic health records (EHRs) merely reflects bias in the culture as a whole in the medical community and bias in the way the health care system is structured. (Lagu)
- The simplest evidence-based practice to improve care for people with disabilities is to provide accommodations for those who need them. (Lagu)
- Disability status needs to be in a prominent place in the EHR to ensure the necessary accommodations are in place for a person's clinical encounter. (Morris)
- Moving forward requires providing evidence-based data to provide disability-friendly care. (Mahmoudi)
- Patients with disabilities say the best thing a provider can do is ask about their disability and any accommodations they need to have a more productive appointment. (Morris)
- Learning to speak respectfully to individuals with disabilities would help improve what clinicians are entering into the EHR. (Warren)
- One issue for individuals going through the disability determination process is the amount of outdated information in an EHR that follows a patient as the years go by and that, while no longer true, still affects both how other clinicians view the

individual and how the disability determination process considers an application. (Price)

The workshop's final session was a discussion moderated by Elham Mahmoudi, planning committee member and associate professor of health economics at the University of Michigan. The final panelists were Megan Morris, Julia Adler-Milstein, V. G. Vinod Vydiswaran, Prerana Laddha, and Tara Lagu. The discussion was limited to the panelists, representatives of the Social Security Administration (SSA), prior speakers, and members of the planning committee.

Mahmoudi's first question for the panel regarded how to address the racism or labelism language in the unstructured fields in the MyChart patient portal embedded in Epic's electronic health record (EHR). Morris replied that the field is early in thinking through bias in EHRs, and most of the work has addressed race and ethnicity. The first thing to do in the disability space, she said, is to define biased language in the context of disability. For example, she hears from family members that they perceive "goals of care" as a veiled way to suggest discontinuing treatment or not starting treatment because of a person's disability. "Once we are able to define it, then we are able to identify it," said Morris. She noted that researchers create interventions in the EHR that alert providers when they use biased language and suggest alternative language.

Lagu added that bias in EHRs merely reflects bias in the culture as a whole in the medical community and bias in the way the health care system is structured. The bigger challenge to her is how to reorient medical education to teach students how to care for people with disabilities, how to talk about people with disabilities, to understand that people with disabilities are everywhere, and to be inclusive not just in the language they use in the EHR, but also in the way they provide care. She said:

> There have been some promising grassroots movements from medical students and trainees, and I would love to see some of that continue because I think we are at a moment when we have the opportunity to change the culture of medicine and the health care system for the better.

Laddha noted the importance of capturing the patient's version of their story, giving them the flexibility to define their situation in their own words, and making that part of the EHR.

CAPTURING FUNCTIONAL INFORMATION

Mahmoudi said as far as he can tell, information about functional status is not currently gathered anywhere. Given that, he wondered how current technology—machine learning, natural language processing (NLP), and artificial intelligence (AI)—could collect this information and make it readily and easily available to providers. Vydiswaran answered that collecting information is not what AI and NLP can do. Rather, somebody must capture that information and document it in the EHR, which is the unsolved problem with its own biases. However, if the information is captured and it is not in a standardized field, that is where NLP, and particularly AI, can help. NLP systems typically start with a keyword-based approach to define what the model needs to capture, but these do not cover all the variations in the English language. This is where AI-based approaches that use context are more efficient and effective, and it is where generative AI approaches are getting better at summarizing information that might be in the clinical documentation. The key is training the AI models with good-quality data, which requires human input to identify factors more representative of the conditions of interest and those that are not, which is equally important.

Morris commented that disability and functional status can be separate concepts. She noted that in the standards the Office of the National Coordinator for Health Information Technology is promulgating, disability status and functional status appear among the health status identifiers, not in the demographics section. However, if the goal is to use the data in the disability determination process, it is imperative to think about who is at risk, and that means identifying the demographics of people who are at risk.

Mahmoudi asked Laddha how the community can advocate to add functional status and functionality to the EHR. Laddha said that when national standards are available, it is easy for a technology vendor to implement a change in a way that is available to every consumer out of the box. Absent standards, the EHR vendor can add flexibility in the software to enable the user to define a version or variation of a standard in a way that is most meaningful to the user's demographic area, health system, or target population. This, she said, is where the work Morris is doing is helpful for technology partners as it serves as a starting point for health systems, absent a national standard, to make their own modifications to their EHR system.

ENABLING BIDIRECTIONAL COMMUNICATION WITH COMMUNITY PARTNERS

Laddha also discussed how health care systems can communicate with community-based services in a format compliant with the Health Insurance

Portability and Accountability Act when the community-based organization is not using the Epic system. Michigan Medicine, for example, had to use Dropbox to serve as an intermediary between the health system and community organizations. Noting there is a great deal of interest in addressing this issue, Laddha said several things need to happen when bringing in community partners and engaging them to help patients. The first is understanding the target population and what assistance they need. "Identify the target population and have the analytics in place that can identify inequities and needs," she said.

The second step is to for the health care system to name a community liaison who will engage with the community. "I do not want to underestimate how difficult that task is, so having a named community liaison that can help you through that process is extremely beneficial," said Laddha. The community liaison, working with others in the health care system, then identifies the appropriate community partners. The third step is to involve the technology partner and take advantage of their open-source application interfaces that community-based organizations can use to create a closed-loop referral system, though Laddha acknowledged that taking this step is still in its infancy. "For [community-benefit organizations] to set up a process where someone is going in electronically and responding to referrals is still a hard task," she said. This is where financial incentives for these community-benefit organizations to do this work can help.

Laddha said her organization has developed a light-weight platform for its Epic system to create closed-loop systems with community partners. In Wisconsin, for example, the company developed this platform for doulas because the health care system thought it beneficial to share more of a patient's history with the doulas to provide the right care.

PROVIDING EVIDENCE-BASED, DISABILITY-FRIENDLY CARE

Following Laddha's comment about incentives for community-based organizations, Mahmoudi wondered if data showed that addressing the social needs of patients, particularly those with disabilities, reduced hospital readmissions, then might it be possible to provide incentives to these community resources? Laddha replied that value-based contracts with providers could work, given payers have shown some interest in funding community-based organizations. Adler-Milstein said this question ties into the challenge of making a case for health systems to invest in disability-friendly care. Unaware of whether the data to make that case exists, she said this would be a good area for study to generate such data. She wondered if it would be possible to articulate a national-scale transformation effort around what disability-friendly health systems would look like that would engage community partners and then design incentives based on that effort. To go along with the incentives, it would be imperative to provide evidence-based care practices that, if followed, would earn those incentives.

Lagu said there is definitely a need for more research to identify evidence-based practices that improve care for people with disabilities. However, there are some practices that work because they have face validity, because patients report they are happier when those practices occur, and because they are best for quality and safety. The simplest practice, she added, is providing accommodations for people who need them.

D'Sena' Warren said the question should not be how to keep people with a disability out of the hospital, but why are they going to the hospital in the first place. Usually, she said, it is because going to the emergency department to receive treatment is better than waiting for six months to two years to get an appointment with a specialist. Lagu said she has data to back up Warren's comment. "We have qualitative data for patients with disabilities who report that they cannot access care, they cannot get appointments with some specialists, and they cannot get the testing they need," said Lagu. "In some cases, it is their physicians who tell them to go to the emergency room because they say, 'You are not going to be able to get this care anywhere but in the hospital.'"

Mahmoudi, agreeing with Laddha, Lagu, and Warren, said moving forward requires providing evidence-based data to provide disability-friendly care. In his opinion, it may be productive to provide data showing that if a health system provides that type of care, it will reduce the costs of readmissions and preventable hospitalizations or emergency department visits in addition to helping their patients have a better quality of life and fewer adverse health events. Morris said she would love to do that research if anyone wants to fund it, something that has been difficult so far. The National Institutes of Health's (NIH) decision to consider individuals with disabilities a disparity population may be a good first step to getting this type of research funded.

Z CODES AND DOCUMENTING SOCIAL DETERMINANTS OF HEALTH

Changing subjects, Mahmoudi asked the panelists for their thoughts on how to use Z codes more efficiently to identify social determinants in a more standardized manner. Adler-Milstein said her health system does not use them, even when clinicians know there is a social need. "I think the issue is some combination of awareness and our clinicians not seeing the value of documenting the codes," she said. "I think it is a helpful step that they exist, but I think we have to be sure that there is some structure to show the value of using them." She also blamed a reluctance to use Z codes for this purpose because of the messiness of the problem list tied to the Z codes and the complexity of deciding what code to use for which social need. "Unfortunately, I just do not think there is a strong case for their use right now," said Adler-Milstein.

Lagu argued the question is not about what diagnostic codes should be in the EHR, but what is the reason for thinking they are even needed. "I think the reasons are that we do not know who has a disability, who needs accommodation, and who has health-related social needs," said Lagu. Her view is to collect the data to identify who has needs and then inform the health systems to provide the services and accommodations to meet those needs.

Laddha noted that Z codes help with interoperability, and Warren added that what she does not like about them is that the names and diagnoses associated with them are always changing. Vydiswaran said Z codes are not meant to be an end-to-end solution. "It is a very specific solution people have come up with that could help with interoperability," he explained. To him, the critical first step is not about documenting disability, but documenting the need for accommodations early, often, and continuously so changes in a person's functional status that occur over time are also recorded. In addition, he emphasized the need to develop a continuous, standardized way of capturing information before thinking that Z codes could be a solution.

IDENTIFYING BIAS

Vincent Nibali asked if there are any indicators to look for in existing EHRs to identify when the information contains biases to adjudicate. Lagu replied that since the EHR is not providing information about who has a disability, spotting biases is difficult. Spotting biased language may be one hint, she said, as could being discharged from a practice, though that can be difficult to determine. Morris noted she and her colleagues completed a randomized controlled trial for which they recruited people with communication-related disabilities. "We came up with 300 ICD10 codes that might have been relevant, and those patients with scheduled appointments with those ICD10 codes were called," said Morris. "About 50 percent of the people who we were able to get ahold of actually denied having a communication-related disability."

Though this study could not answer the question of why people did not identify as having a disability, what it indicated was that ICD10 codes have problems. "I think the message is coming across: We need to ask," said Morris. Once people are asked and that information is in the EHR, it might be possible to find indications in the medical notes that could identify these individuals. "There might not be. I think we have to be prepared for that," Morris said. Lagu added that it is important to ask about accommodations too.

Warren, who said she has dealt with physician bias throughout her journey of applying for disability, had a note in her chart from her neurologist that contradicted what he told her. She appealed and was told that changing the EHR was up to her neurologist, and he would change his notes. However, her EHR noted her appeal and that, together with a wealth of other information she supplied to Social Security, led to her disability determination being approved.

Lagu said that there are certain health systems that do better at avoiding bias toward people with disabilities, including rehabilitation hospitals and stroke rehabilitation facilities. Children's hospitals have advanced methods of dealing with people with developmental disabilities. These systems could provide valuable lessons about best practices, she said. Vydiswaran commented that research has shown the doctor–patient dyad has a significant role in determining whether information in the EHR is biased.

Amy J. Houtrow, noting that medical students and residents are now being trained not to mention someone's race or ethnicity in their notes, asked the panelists for their thoughts about how to appropriately include information in the EHR in a manner that best serves people with disabilities and does not further perpetuate discrimination against them, especially for those with an invisible disability that might not be readily apparent at a first encounter. Morris replied that even if clinicians are being instructed not to include that information in their notes, it is still in the EHR as part of the demographic information. To her, disability status needs to be in a prominent place in the EHR to ensure the necessary accommodations are in place for a person's clinical encounter. Mahmoudi noted that when he and his colleagues contacted individuals in wheelchairs because of a spinal cord injury, the individuals did not want to be labeled as someone with a disability because they felt they were not disabled. Instead, they wanted to be identified as a person with a spinal cord injury.

ABOVE ALL, ASK

Morris recounted the findings of a study she and her collaborators conducted in which they had medical students come into a standardized clinical scenario after randomizing them to either have or not have a person with a disability as their patient. The student noticed the disability but did not ask the patient about it because they assumed the patient would be ashamed of their disability and bringing it up would make them feel bad. However, what she has heard repeatedly from patients with disabilities is that the best thing a provider can do is ask, about both the disability and any accommodations they need to have a more productive appointment. Lagu noted that providers now ask about the pronouns people use, so in the same vein, they should ask about disabilities. She added there are web pages with information on basic disability etiquette, and that all clinicians would benefit from learning basic disability etiquette so they could speak to people with disabilities in the way they want to be addressed. Mahmoudi agreed there is a need for more education for all medical professionals on how to talk about sensitive subjects with their patients, and Lagu said the accreditation bodies that oversee medical education need to take this up as an important issue.

IMPROVING THE DISABILITY DETERMINATION PROCESS

Lagu raised the issue of how SSA could improve the disability determination process to make it more accessible to the community it serves. She said things she took away from the workshop were the importance of collecting data and the need to educate clinicians on how to document their patients' disabilities in the EHR. She applauded Yvonne M. Perret for her approach of compiling a holistic picture of her patients that incorporates social determinants, medical issues, and other crises they face and putting that in the EHR so it can be considered in the determination process. "I just wonder why there are not more Yvonnes out there and why our system is not supporting more people who do this for vulnerable patients," said Lagu.

Adler-Milstein said what struck her is that everyone feels they provide a great deal of information and fill out many forms. "It is not like there are no opportunities to collect information from people," she said. She wondered if there is a need to step back and look for the touch points at which to best collect the most information most efficiently in a manner that would engender trust. She noted that Medicaid enrollment is taking this approach to identify natural opportunities to catch people when they first move.

Vydiswaran said that educating future clinicians early in their training about documenting disabilities and social needs is important, but SSA should also recognize that biases exist and that they are probably playing a role in how clinicians are documenting disabilities in the medical record. Recognizing that and looking at the entire package of what patients are saying and significantly enhancing their voices in the process would help too. This is where training those making these determinations about bias would help.

Warren said learning to speak respectfully to individuals with disabilities would help improve what clinicians are entering into the EHR, and Morris highlighted the need to think about access to the disability determination process given the challenge people with disabilities have with getting to a disability determination hearing or appointment. She also noted that this process can hurt the patient–provider relationship because of the onerous amount of paperwork a provider must complete for their patient.

Amanda Price, from NIH, said one issue for individuals going through the disability determination process is the amount of outdated information in an EHR that follows a patient as the years go by and that, while no longer true, still affects both how other clinicians view the individual and how the disability determination process considers an application.

THE ROLE OF AI

Mahmoudi asked the panelists for their thoughts on the use of AI in the health care system. Vydiswaran replied that AI is not a solution, just a means to an end. In his view, AI should *not* be used to create a persona of what a patient is, and that persona should not be put in the EHR to serve as a summary of what the health system thinks about the patient. He noted Warren's issue with contesting a statement in her EHR from her neurologist and wondered if the situation would be the same for an AI-generated statement. "I would caution against using AI as a replacement for what the health system thinks about the patient," said Vydiswaran. It would be important, too, to use the appropriate training data to avoid biased results from an AI-powered process.

Adler-Milstein said AI is not ready to make disability determinations, but it could help humans be more efficient so they have more time to have the necessary discussions. One thing AI can do well is access a much larger pool of information to see relevant signals in the EHR that are now overlooked, though as Price noted, there can be misleading and outdated information in the EHR. Joy Amaryllis Johnson added that AI might be a problem for a community that does not know about it because her clients are suspicious of new technology.

Jonathan Platt commented that people are now aware that AI can be biased, and he wondered if that knowledge can be used to train clinicians to use language that is less biased. Kenrick Cato said that AI does a good job of capturing the demographic-level bias in the workflow of health care, so AI systems today will give answers that are biased. Adler-Milstein said the question for AI systems is what the acceptable level of precision is versus the efficiency gains that might result from using an AI model to extract information from the EHR.

THE IMPORTANCE OF TRUST

Speaking of trust, Adler-Milstein, responding to Johnson's question about the role of insurance companies in this process, said she is inclined to say that insurers have a significant role to play in solving the problems raised at the workshop, but are the least trusted entity in the health care system, according to consumers. That is why she has been hesitant to involve insurers.

Morris said there is not enough conversation about the mistrust the disability community has in the medical establishment. "There is a long history of abuses in the United States against people with disabilities, especially in medicine, and we have not recognized that and acknowledged how entering into the health care system can be retraumatizing for these individuals," she said. "We need to think about building our trust with our community of individuals with disabilities." As a final comment to conclude the workshop, Houtrow said the big message from the discussions is to include people with disabilities at all steps of the process.

10

Concluding Remarks

Amy J. Houtrow provided a summary of the main messages from the two days of presentations and discussion. She began by reinforcing the message articulated by multiple panelists that people with disabilities face discriminatory forces and multiple barriers to care. Further, such discrimination and access barriers can have serious detrimental consequences to their health and well-being. In addition to disability discrimination, or ableism, disabled individuals often also have other oppressed identities, such as being minoritized (facing racism) and facing classism, including the experience of being unhoused.

As explained by Jonathan Platt on the first day of the workshop, social and political determinants of health, which are the main drivers of health, are the conditions into which we are born, live, learn, love, work, and play. These determinants of health are maintained by mutually reinforcing systems of both opportunity and oppression in the housing, financing, employment, health care, and criminal justice systems. Houtrow noted that although it is possible to make changes to the social determinants of health, such change is hard. In health care, there is often a disconnect between what is provided and what people need to be as healthy as possible.

Houtrow reinforced what the lived expertise panelists explained about how challenging it is to navigate the numerous areas of the health care system and how it feels to try to do so while facing discrimination by health care providers. Houtrow observed, "It was hard for me to hear…that there is incredible disrespect, denial, and dismissal of people with disabilities when they try to access the care they need and that they deserve." Patients may be dismissed by their providers or deemed to be angry or to be overemphasizing their symptoms. Others may miss an appointment because they do not have adequate transportation or may have some emergency that needs to be prioritized, yet health care providers say these individuals are "no-shows," which gets incorporated into their medical chart and creates a bias in how they are understood by health care providers moving forward. Similarly, other data that is inaccurate may be incorporated into and then perpetuated in a person's medical record.

Experts have clearly stated that capturing a patient's story in their own words is tremendously important, but even then, providers may introduce bias. Houtrow provided an example: "Jane Doe alleges 10 out of 10 pain, saying this is the worst pain I have ever felt in my life, versus, John Doe has 10 out of 10 pain and says this is the worst pain I have ever experienced in my life." The term *alleges* in the first sentence introduces bias language into the record. It tells people that the provider does not necessarily believe that that individual is reporting accurately on their pain. Houtrow said, "Bias exists in medical records because health care providers are biased, because systems are biased, because society is biased against people with disabilities."

Houtrow reiterated what panelists reported in terms of the challenges people face in navigating the Social Security Administration's (SSA's) disability determination processes. Some individuals experience data poverty in their medical records, making the determination process more challenging. People who are marginalized often have less accurate and less valuable data in the medical record. They also might have less data overall because of the barriers they experience in accessing care. When people with disabilities are denied the care they need, it is difficult for them to get the information they need into their medical record so they can successfully go through the disability determination process. As panelists reported, it is also hard for them to trust the health care system. This makes the disability community worried at times about sharing their data and may drive them to seek care in places outside of traditional health care settings. The medical system needs to earn back that trust of people with disabilities.

Academic experts, experts who are working in the community, and people with lived expertise shared ideas for change and structural and policy reforms, including incentives and training for doctors; expanding who can do consultative examinations, how they are done, and sources from which information is gathered; and the need to simplify the disability determination process to make it easier for people to go through it. Houtrow noted the importance of this because doctors and other health care professionals feel burdened by the paperwork necessary for the disability determinations. She identified the importance of supporting the work of people working in communities of need as well as the value of having a provider who reflects oneself and one's culture, noting the need for a lot of workforce development.

With respect to electronic health records (EHRs), speakers conveyed a great passion for collecting data about disability in the medical record and the need to make it easy to collect such data and to have it be accurate and up-to-date because disability and people's health needs change over time. Capturing the determinants of health in the Epic EHR system can help promote engagement between provider and patient. In addition to making sure providers are addressing someone's disability needs, EHRs can assist providers in making referrals for other services, such as Meals on Wheels, and by providing potential options for supports and resources.

Disability status may be self-reported as an identity or a demographic characteristic. EHRs can also capture an individual's functional limitations and the accommodations they need, but there need to be strategies to collect these data prior to medical appointments so patients can have their needs met through accommodations at the time they are seeking care. Additionally, panelists expressed the importance of using tools that are validated, but such tools do not guarantee an accurate reflection of individual experiences. As noted previously, biases can be incorporated into the medical record, and there is a disconnect between how doctors and other health care providers think about the history captured in a medical record and what SSA considers to be objective medical evidence in the health record.

Despite their promises, EHRs also bring challenges. EHR systems differ across health care systems. Not all systems are able to exchange information with one another, although the ideal would be to have HIPAA-compliant interoperability among medical record systems. In addition, some systems cost more than others. Some provider groups, such as federally qualified health centers (FQHCs), have fewer resources to spend on EHRs, which sets up a kind of digital divide. When the patients who are served by these FQHCs are the same people who face oppressive forces and lack of access to the things they need, they face an additional disparity in which even their medical record systems are less robust than the ones that typically exist in academic medical centers. Furthermore, patients with disabilities and other oppressed identities tend to have less access to the patient portals. In addition to language and cultural differences, the portals are not always disability accessible. Such digital barriers can actually worsen disparities for already disadvantaged groups.

New ways of collecting, accessing, viewing, understanding, aggregating, and analyzing health data are evolving, and there may be a future in which artificial intelligence (AI) will help these processes become more efficient and provide analysis of many more pieces of information. Policy can drive behavior in capturing data, and health care professionals need to be educated around appropriate documentation as well as in providing care for people with disabilities.

Houtrow concluded by observing that the most important message is to do the following:

> Include people with disabilities. "Nothing about us without us." Respect the expertise of people with disabilities, listen to them, believe them, and truly engage them. That's engaging them in the design of, the development of, the implementation of, the evaluation of programs, services, policies, and the like.

Alongside the importance of engaging people with disabilities are the importance of addressing biases and especially of having data to inform processes, strategies, and treatment in a way that helps reduce disparities and improve care and outcomes for people with disabilities.

Appendix A

References

Adler-Milstein, J., A. J. Holmgren, P. Kralovec, C. Worzala, T. Searcy, and V. Patel. 2017. Electronic health record adoption in US hospitals: The emergence of a digital "advanced use" divide. *Journal of the American Medical Informatics Association* 24(6):1142–1148. https://doi.org/10.1093/jamia/ocx080.

Bezyak, J. L., S. Sabella, J. Hammel, K. McDonald, R. A. Jones, and D. Barton. 2020. Community participation and public transportation barriers experienced by people with disabilities. *Disability and Rehabilitation* 42(23):3275–3283. https://doi.org/10.1080/09638288.2019.1590469.

Bixby, L., S. Bevan, and C. Boen. 2022. The links between disability, incarceration, and social exclusion. *Health Affairs* 41(10):1460–1469. https://doi.org/10.1377/hlthaff.2022.00495.

Boyd, A. D., R. Gonzalez-Guarda, K. Lawrence, C. L. Patil, M. O. Ezenwa, E. C., O'Brien, H. Paek, J. M. Braciszewski, O. Adeyemi, A. M. Cuthel, J. E. Darby, C. K. Zigler, P. M. Ho, K. R. Faurot, K. Staman, J. W. Leigh, D. L. Dailey, A. Cheville, G. Del Fiol, M. R. Knisely, K. Marsolo, R. L. Richesson, and J. M. Schlaeger. 2023a. Equity and bias in electronic health records data. *Contemporary Clinical Trials* 130(July):107238. https://doi.org/10.1016/j.cct.2023.107238.

Boyd, A. D., R. Gonzalez-Guarda, K. Lawrence, C. L. Patil, M. O. Ezenwa, E. C., O'Brien, H. Paek, J. M. Braciszewski, O. Adeyemi, A. M. Cuthel, J. E. Darby, C. K. Zigler, P. M. Ho, K. R. Faurot, K. Staman, J. W. Leigh, D. L. Dailey, A. Cheville, G. Del Fiol, M. R. Knisely, C. R. Grudzen, K. Marsolo, R. L. Richesson, and J. M. Schlaeger. 2023b. Potential bias and lack of generalizability in electronic health record data: Reflections on health equity from the National Institutes of Health Pragmatic Trials Collaboratory. *Journal of the American Medical Informatics Association* 30(9):1561–1566. https://doi.org/10.1093/jamia/ocad115.

Bradshaw, R. L., K. Kawamoto, J. R. Bather, M. S. Goodman, W. K. Kohlmann, D. Chavez-Yenter, M. Volkmar, R. Monahan, K. A. Kaphingst, and G. Del Fiol. 2024. Enhanced family history-based algorithms increase the identification of individuals meeting criteria for genetic testing of hereditary cancer syndromes but would not reduce disparities on their own. *Journal of Biomedical Informatics* 149(January):104–568. https://doi.org/10.1016/j.jbi.2023.104568.

Bright, T. J., A. Wong, R. Dhurjati, E. Bristow, L. Bastian, R. R. Coeytaux, G. Samsa, V. Hasselblad, J. W. Williams, M. D. Musty, L. Wing, A. S. Kendrick, G. D. Sanders, and D. Lobach. 2012. Effect of clinical decision-support systems. *Annals of Internal Medicine* 157(1):29–43. https://doi.org/10.7326/0003-4819-157-1-201207030-00450.

Brown, E. M., S. M. Franklin, J. L. Ryan, M. Canterberry, A. Bowe, M. S. Pantell, E. K. Cottrell, and L. M. Gottlieb. 2023. Assessing area-level deprivation as a proxy for individual-level social risks. *American Journal of Preventive Medicine* 65(6):1163–1171. https://doi.org/10.1016/j.amepre.2023.06.006.

Budd, J. 2023. Burnout related to electronic health record use in primary care. *Journal of Primary Care & Community Health* 14. https://doi.org/10.1177/21501319231166921.

Buis, L. R., L. K. Brown, M. A. Plegue, R. Kadri, A. R. Laurie, T. C. Guetterman, V. G. V. Vydiswaran, J. Li, and T. C. Veinot. 2023. Identifying inequities in video and audio telehealth services for primary care encounters during COVID-19: Repeated cross-sectional, observational study. *Journal of Medical Internet Research* 25:e49804. https://doi.org/10.2196/49804.

Calandra, L., P. Camilla, S. Abi, and T. K. Daniel. 2022. Electronic medical record-related burnout in healthcare providers: A scoping review of outcomes and interventions. *BMJ Open* 12(8):e060865. https://doi.org/10.1136/bmjopen-2022-060865.

Casau, A., and M. C. Beach. 2022. *Words matter: Strategies to reduce bias in electronic health records.* https://www.chcs.org/media/Words-Matter-Strategies-to-Reduce-Bias-in-Electronic-Health-Records_102022.pdf (accessed June 13, 2024).

CDC (U.S. Centers for Disease Control and Prevention). 2024. *Disability and health overview.* https://www.cdc.gov/ncbddd/disabilityandhealth/disability.html (accessed June 13, 2024).

Chang, W., and C. Richwine. 2023. *Social needs screening among non-federal acute care hospitals, 2022.* https://www.healthit.gov/sites/default/files/2023-07/Social_Needs_Screening_among_Non-Federal_Acute_Care_Hospitals_2022-508.pdf (accessed June 13, 2024).

Chavez-Yenter, D., M. S. Goodman, Y. Chen, X. Chu, R. L. Bradshaw, R. Lorenz Chambers, P. A. Chan, B. M. Daly, M. Flynn, A. Gammon, R. Hess, C. Kessler, W. K. Kohlmann, D. M. Mann, R. Monahan, S. Peel, K. Kawamoto, G. Del Fiol, M. Sigireddi, S. S. Buys, O. Ginsburg, and K. A. Kaphingst. 2022. Association of disparities in family history and family cancer history in the electronic health record with sex, race, Hispanic or Latino ethnicity, and language preference in 2 large US health care systems. *JAMA Network Open* 5(10):e2234574. https://doi.org/10.1001/jamanetworkopen.2022.34574.

Chen, Z., N. Liang, H. Zhang, H. Li, Y. Yang, X. Zong, Y. Chen, Y. Wang, and N. Shi. 2023. Harnessing the power of clinical decision support systems: Challenges and opportunities. *Open Heart* 10(2):e002432. https://doi.org/10.1136/openhrt-2023-002432.

Chin, M. H., N. Afsar-Manesh, A. S. Bierman, C. Chang, C. J. Colón-Rodríguez, P. Dullabh, D. G. Duran, M. Fair, T. Hernandez-Boussard, M. Hightower, A. Jain, W. B. Jordan, S. Konya, R. H. Moore, T. T. Moore, R. Rodriguez, G. Shaheen, L. P. Snyder, M. Srinivasan, C. A. Umschied, and L. Ohno-Machado. 2023. Guiding principles to address the impact of algorithm bias on racial and ethnic disparities in health and health care. *JAMA Network Open* 6(12):e2345050. https://doi.org/10.1001/jamanetworkopen.2023.45050.

Civil Rights Division. 2008. *Americans with Disabilities Act of 1990, as amended*. U.S. Department of Justice. https://www.ada.gov/law-and-regs/ada/ (accessed June 13, 2024).

Coleman-Jensen, A. 2020. U.S. food insecurity and population trends with a focus on adults with disabilities. *Physiology and Behavior* 220(June):112865. https://doi.org/10.1016/j.physbeh.2020.112865.

Coleman, K. J., C. Stewart, B. E. Waitzfelder, J. E. Zeber, L. S. Morales, A. T. Ahmed, B. K. Ahmedani, A. Beck, L. A. Copeland, J. R. Cummings, E. M. Hunkeler, N. M. Lindberg, F. Lynch, C. Y. Lu, A. A. Owen-Smith, C. M. Trinacty, R. R. Whitebird, and G. E. Simon. 2016. Racial-ethnic differences in psychiatric diagnoses and treatment across 11 health care systems in the mental health research network. *Psychiatric Services* 67(7):749–757. https://doi.org/10.1176/appi.ps.201500217.

Connor, D. J., and B. A. Ferri. 2005. Integration and inclusion: A troubling nexus: Race, disability, and special education. *Journal of African American History* 90(1/2):107–127. http://www.jstor.org/stable/20063978 (accessed June 13, 2024).

Cook, L. A., J. Sachs, and N. G. Weiskopf. 2021. The quality of social determinants data in the electronic health record: A systematic review. *Journal of American Medical Informatics Association* 29(1):187–196. https://doi.org/10.1093/jamia/ocab199.

Cottrell, E. K., M. Hendricks, K. Dambrun, S. Cowburn, M. Pantell, R. Gold, and L. M. Gottlieb. 2020. Comparison of community-level and patient-level social risk data in a network of community health centers. *JAMA Network Open* 3(10):e2016852. https://doi.org/10.1001/jamanetworkopen.2020.16852.

de Groot, A. C. 2020. Fragrances: Contact allergy and other adverse effects. *Dermatitis* 31(1):13–35. https://doi.org/10.1097/der.0000000000000463.

Evans, W. N., and C. L. Garthwaite. 2014. Giving mom a break: The impact of higher EITC payments on maternal health. *American Economic Journal* 6(2):258–290. https://doi.org/10.1257/pol.6.2.258.

Gallo, K. P., and D. H. Barlow. 2012. Factors involved in clinician adoption and nonadoption of evidence-based interventions in mental health. *Clinical Psychology: Science and Practice* 19(1):93–106. https://doi.org/10.1111/j.1468-2850.2012.01276.x.

Gómez, C. A., D. V. Kleinman, N. Pronk, G. L. Wrenn Gordon, E. Ochiai, C. Blakey, A. Johnson, and K. H. Brewer. 2021. Addressing health equity and social determinants of health through Healthy People 2030. *Journal of Public Health Management and Practice* 27(Supplement 6):S249–S257. https://journals.lww.com/jphmp/fulltext/2021/11001/addressing_health_equity_and_social_determinants.9.aspx (accessed June 13, 2024).

Han, H.-R., K. T. Gleason, C.-A. Sun, H. N. Miller, S. J. Kang, S. Chow, R. Anderson, P. Nagy, P., and T. Bauer. 2019. Using patient portals to improve patient outcomes: Systematic review. *JMIR Human Factors* 6(4):e15038. https://doi.org/10.2196/15038.

Harper, S., N. B. King, S. C. Meersman, M. E. Reichman, N. Breen, and J. Lynch. 2010. Implicit value judgments in the measurement of health inequalities. *The Milbank Quarterly* 88(1):4–29. https://doi.org/10.1111/j.1468-0009.2010.00587.x.

Holder, M., H. B. Waldman, and H. Hood. 2009. Preparing health professionals to provide care to individuals with disabilities. *International Journal of Oral Science* 1(2):66–71. https://doi.org/10.4248/ijos.09022.

Ibrahim, H., X. Liu, N. Zariffa, A. D. Morris, and A. K. Denniston. 2021. Health data poverty: An assailable barrier to equitable digital health care. *The Lancet Digital Health* 3(4):e260–e265. https://doi.org/10.1016/s2589-7500(20)30317-4.

Iezzoni, L. I., S. R. Rao, J. Ressalam, D. Bolcic-Jankovic, N. D. Agaronnik, K. Donelan, T. Lagu, and E. G. Campbell. 2021. Physicians' perceptions of people with disability and their health care. *Health Affairs (Millwood)* 40(2):297–306. https://doi.org/10.1377/hlthaff.2020.01452.

Iezzoni, L. I., S. R. Rao, J. Ressalam, D. Bolcic-Jankovic, N. D. Agaronnik, T. Lagu, E. Pendo, and E. G. Campbell. 2022. US physicians' knowledge about The Americans with Disabilities Act and accommodation of patients with disability. *Health Affairs (Millwood)*. 2022 41(1):96–104. https://doi.org/10.1377/hlthaff.2021.01136.

Institute of Medicine. 2014a. *Capturing social and behavioral domains and measures in electronic health records: Phase 2*. Washington, DC: The National Academies Press. https://doi.org/10.17226/18951.

Institute of Medicine. 2014b. *Capturing social and behavioral domains in electronic health records: Phase 1*. Washington, DC: The National Academies Press. https://doi.org/10.17226/18709.

Iott, B. E., M. S. Pantell, J. Adler-Milstein, and L. M. Gottlieb. 2022. Physician awareness of social determinants of health documentation capability in the electronic health record. *Journal of the American Medical Informatics Association* 29(12):2110–2116. https://doi.org/10.1093/jamia/ocac154.

Iott, B. E., J. Adler-Milstein, L. M. Gottlieb, and M. S. Pantell. 2023. Characterizing the relative frequency of clinician engagement with structured social determinants of health data. *Journal of the American Medical Informatics Association* 30(3):503–510. https://doi.org/10.1093/jamia/ocac251.

Iott, B. E., L. Samantha Rivas, L. M. Gottlieb, J. Adler-Milstein, M. S. Pantell. 2024. Structured and unstructured social risk factor documentation in the electronic health record underestimates patients' self-reported risks. *Journal of the American Medical Informatics Association* 31(3):714–719. https://doi.org/10.1093/jamia/ocad261.

Jones, C. P. 2000. Levels of racism: A theoretic framework and a gardener's tale. *American Journal of Public Health* 90(8):1212–1215. https://doi.org/10.2105/ajph.90.8.1212.

Kan, K., C. Foster, B. Orionzi, D. Schinasi, and N. Heard-Garris. 2024. More than one divide: A multilevel view of the digital determinants of health. *Journal of Pediatrics* 266:113820. https://doi.org/10.1016/j.jpeds.2023.113820.

Kaphingst, K. A., W. Kohlmann, R. L. Chambers, M. S. Goodman, R. Bradshaw, P. A. Chan, D. Chavez-Yenter, S. V. Colonna, W. F. Espinel, J. N. Everett, A. Gammon, E. Goldberg, R. J. Gonzalez, K. J. Hagerty, R. Hess, K. Kehoe, C. Kessler, K. E. Kimball, S. Loomis, T. R. Martinez, R. Monahan, J. D. Schiffman, D. Temares, K. Tobik, D. W. Wetter, D. M. Mann, K. Kawamoto, G. Del Fiol, S. S. Buys, and O. Ginsburg. 2021. Comparing models of delivery for cancer genetics services among patients receiving primary care who meet criteria for genetic evaluation in two healthcare systems: BRIDGE randomized controlled trial. *BMC Health Services Research* 21(1):542. https://doi.org/10.1186/s12913-021-06489-y.

Kawamoto, K., M. C. Flynn, P. Kukhareva, D. ElHalta, R. Hess, T. Gregory, C. Walls, A. M. Wigren, D. Borbolla, B. E. Bray, M. H. Parsons, B. L. Clayson, M. S. Briley, C. H. Stipelman, D. Taylor, C. S. King, G. Del Fiol, T. J. Reese, C. R. Weir, T. Taft, and M. B. Strong. 2018. A pragmatic guide to establishing clinical decision support governance and addressing decision support fatigue: A case study. *AMIA Annual Symposium Proceedings* 2018:624–633.

Krahn, G. L., D. K. Walker, and R. Correa-De-Araujo. 2015. Persons with disabilities as an unrecognized health disparity population. *American Journal of Public Health* 105(Supplement 2):S198–S206. https://doi.org/10.2105/ajph.2014.302182.

Krieger, N. 2001. A glossary for social epidemiology. *Journal of Epidemiology and Community Health* 55(10):693–700. https://doi.org/10.1136/jech.55.10.693.

Kruse, C. S., C. Kristof, B. Jones, E. Mitchell, and A. Martinez. 2016. Barriers to electronic health record adoption: A systematic literature review. *Journal of Medical Systems* 40(12):252. https://doi.org/10.1007/s10916-016-0628-9.

Lagu, T., N. S. Hannon, M. B. Rothberg, A. S. Wells, K. L. Green, M. O. Windom, K. R. Dempsey, P. S. Pekow, J. S. Avrunin, A. Chen, A., and P. K. Lindenauer. 2013. Access to subspecialty care for patients with mobility impairment: A survey. *Annals of Internal Medicine* 158(6):441–446. https://doi.org/10.7326/0003-4819-158-6-201303190-00003.

Lagu, T., L. I. Iezzoni, and P. K. Lindenauer. 2014. The axes of access—Improving care for patients with disabilities. *New England Journal of Medicine* 370(19):1847–1851. https://doi.org/10.1056/NEJMsb1315940.

Lagu, T., C. Haywood, K. Reimold, C. DeJong, R. Walker Sterling, and L. I. Iezzoni. 2022. 'I am not the doctor for you': Physicians' attitudes about caring for people with disabilities. *Health Affairs (Millwood)* 41(10):1387–1395. https://doi.org/10.1377/hlthaff.2022.00475.

Lybarger, K., O. J. Bear Don't Walk, M. Yetisgen, and Ö. Uzuner. 2023a. Advancements in extracting social determinants of health information from narrative text. *Journal of the American Medical Informatics Association* 30(8):1363–1366. https://doi.org/10.1093/jamia/ocad121.

Lybarger, K., M. Yetisgen, and Ö. Uzuner. 2023b. The 2022 n2c2/UW shared task on extracting social determinants of health. *Journal of the American Medical Informatics Association* 30(8):1367–1378. https://doi.org/10.1093/jamia/ocad012.

Marzolf, B. A., M. A. Plegue, O. Okanlami, D. Meyer, and D. M. Harper. 2022. Are medical students adequately trained to care for persons with disabilities? *PRiMER* 6:34. https://doi.org/10.22454/PRiMER.2022.878147.

Meschede, T., K. Trivedi, and J. Caldwell. 2023. Severe housing and neighborhood inequities of households with disabled members and households in need of long-term services and supports. *Housing and Society* 50(2):228–251. https://doi.org/10.1080/08882746.2022.2065614.

Meseguer, J. 2013. Outcome variation in the Social Security Disability Insurance program: The role of primary diagnoses. *Social Security Bulletin* 73(2):39–75.

Mitra, M., L. M. Long-Bellil, L. I. Iezzoni, S. C. Smeltzer, and L. D. Smith. 2016. Pregnancy among women with physical disabilities: Unmet needs and recommendations on navigating pregnancy. *Disability Health Journal* 9(3):457–463. https://doi.org/10.1016/j.dhjo.2015.12.007.

Mitra, M., I. Akobirshoev, A. Valentine, H. K. Brown, and T. A. Moore Simas. 2021. Severe maternal morbidity and maternal mortality in women with intellectual and developmental disabilities. *American Journal of Preventive Medicine* 61(6):872–881. https://doi.org/10.1016/j.amepre.2021.05.041.

Mitra, M., L. Long-Bellil, I. Moura, A. Miles, and H. S. Kaye. 2022. Advancing health equity and reducing health disparities for people with disabilities in the United States. *Health Affairs (Millwood)* 41(10):1379–1386. https://doi.org/10.1377/hlthaff.2022.00499.

Mitra, M., I. Akobirshoev, A. Valentine, K. McKee, and M. M. McKee. 2024. Severe maternal morbidity in deaf or hard of hearing women in the United States. *Preventive Medicine* 180:107883. https://doi.org/10.1016/j.ypmed.2024.107883.

Morris, A., and C. Alcantara. 2023. Are you ableist? *Washington Post* (April 12). https://www.washingtonpost.com/wellness/interactive/2023/ableist-thinking-disability-bias-quiz/ (accessed June 13, 2024).

Morris, M. A., A. C. Maragh-Bass, J. M. Griffin, L. J. Finney Rutten, T. Lagu, and S. Phelan. 2017. Use of accessible examination tables in the primary care setting: A survey of physical evaluations and patient attitudes. *Journal of General Internal Medicine* 32(12):1342–1348. https://doi.org/10.1007/s11606-017-4155-2.

Morris, Z. A., S. V. McGarity, N. Goodman, and A. Zaidi. 2021. The extra costs associated with living with a disability in the United States. *Journal of Disability Policy Studies* 33(3):158–167. https://doi.org/10.1177/10442073211043521.

National Academy of Medicine. 2017. *Optimizing strategies for clinical decision support: Summary of a meeting series.* Washington, DC: The National Academies Press. https://doi.org/10.17226/27122.

Nowicki, J. M. 2018. *Discipline disparities for Black students, boys, and students with disabilities.* https://www.gao.gov/products/gao-18-258 (accessed June 13, 2024).

Obermeyer, Z., B. Powers, C. Vogeli, and S. Mullainathan. 2019. Dissecting racial bias in an algorithm used to manage the health of populations. *Science* 366(6464):447–453. https://doi.org/10.1126/science.aax2342.

Office of Disability Employment Policy. 2024. *Disability employment statistics.* Department of Labor. https://www.dol.gov/agencies/odep/research-evaluation/statistics (accessed June 13, 2024).

O'Loughlin, K., E. K. Donovan, Z. Radcliff, M. Ryan, and B. Rybarczyk. 2019. Using integrated behavioral healthcare to address behavioral health disparities in underserved populations. *Translational Issues in Psychological Science* 5(4):374–389. https://doi.org/10.1037/tps0000213.

ONC (Office of the National Coordinator for Health Information Technology). 2021a. *National trends in hospital and physician adoption of electronic health records.* https://www.healthit.gov/data/quickstats/national-trends-hospital-and-physician-adoption-electronic-health-records (accessed June 13, 2024).

ONC. 2021b. *Office-based physician electronic health record adoption.* https://www.healthit.gov/data/quickstats/office-based-physician-electronic-health-record-adoption (accessed June 13, 2024).

Peterson, A., V. Charles, D. Yeung, and K. Coyle. 2021. The Health equity framework: A science- and justice-based model for public health researchers and practitioners. *Health Promotion Practice* 22(6):741–746. https://doi.org/10.1177/1524839920950730.

Purpose Built Communities. 2024. *Explore our network by state.* https://purposebuiltcommunities.org/our-network/ (accessed June 13, 2024).

Rajkomar, A., M. Hardt, M. D. Howell, G. Corrado, and M. H. Chin. 2018. Ensuring fairness in machine learning to advance health equity. *Annals of Internal Medicine* 169(12):866–872. https://doi.org/10.7326/m18-1990.

Reed, N. S., L. M. Meeks, and B. K. Swenor. 2020. Disability and COVID-19: Who counts depends on who is counted. *Lancet Public Health* 5(8):e423. https://doi.org/10.1016/s2468-2667(20)30161-4.

Robertson, S. L., M. D. Robinson, and A. Reid. 2017. Electronic health record effects on work-life balance and burnout within the I^3 population collaborative. *Journal of Graduate Medical Education* 9(4):479–484. https://doi.org/10.4300/jgme-d-16-00123.1.

Rowan, A. B., J. Grove, L. Solfelt, and A. Magnante. 2021. Reducing the impacts of mental health stigma through integrated primary care: An examination of the evidence. *Journal of Clinical Psychology in Medical Settings* 28(4):679–693. https://doi.org/10.1007/s10880-020-09742-4.

Roy, L., A. G. Crocker, T. L. Nicholls, E. A. Latimer, and A. R. Ayllon. 2014. Criminal behavior and victimization among homeless individuals with severe mental illness: A systematic review. *Psychiatric Services* 65(6):739–750. https://doi.org/10.1176/appi.ps.201200515.

Saeed, S. A., and R. M. Masters. 2021. Disparities in health care and the digital divide. *Current Psychiatry Reports* 23(9):61. https://doi.org/10.1007/s11920-021-01274-4.

Scheuner, M. T., T. S. McNeel, and A. N. Freedman. 2010. Population prevalence of familial cancer and common hereditary cancer syndromes. The 2005 California Health Interview Survey. *Genetics in Medicine* 12(11):726–735. https://doi.org/10.1097/GIM.0b013e3181f30e9e.

Schwartz, R. C., and D. M. Blankenship. 2014. Racial disparities in psychotic disorder diagnosis: A review of empirical literature. *World Journal of Psychiatry* 4(4):133–140. https://doi.org/10.5498/wjp.v4.i4.133.

Shi, C., M. Goodall, J. Dumville, J. Hill, G. Norman, O. Hamer, A. Clegg, C. L. Watkins, G. Georgiou, A. Hodkinson, C. E. Lightbody, P. Dark, and N. Cullum. 2022. The accuracy of pulse oximetry in measuring oxygen saturation by levels of skin pigmentation: A systematic review and meta-analysis. *BMC Medicine* 20(1):267. https://doi.org/10.1186/s12916-022-02452-8.

Sieck, C. J., A. Sheon, J. S. Ancker, J. Castek, B. Callahan, and A. Siefer. 2021. Digital inclusion as a social determinant of health. *NPJ Digital Medicine* 4(1):52. https://doi.org/10.1038/s41746-021-00413-8.

TAC (Technical Assistance Collaborative). 2014. *Priced out: The housing crisis for people with disabilities.* https://www.tacinc.org/resources/priced-out/ (accessed June 13, 2024).

Urban Institute. 2024. *Disability equity policy.* https://www.urban.org/research-area/disability-equity-policy (accessed June 13, 2024).

Vanderminden, J., and J. J. Esala. 2018. Beyond symptoms: Race and gender predict anxiety disorder diagnosis. *Society and Mental Health* 9(1):111–125. https://doi.org/10.1177/2156869318811435.

Varadaraj, V., J. A. Deal, J. Campanile, N. S. Reed, and B. K. Swenor. 2021. National prevalence of disability and disability types among adults in the US, 2019. *JAMA Network Open* 4(10):e2130358. https://doi.org/10.1001/jamanetworkopen.2021.30358.

Vyas, D. A., L. G. Eisenstein, and D. S. Jones. 2020. Hidden in plain sight—Reconsidering the use of race correction in clinical algorithms. *New England Journal of Medicine* 383(9):874–882. https://doi.org/10.1056/NEJMms2004740.

Vydiswaran, V. G. V., A. Strayhorn, K. Weber, H. Stevens, J. Mellinger, G. S. Winder, and A. C. Fernandez. 2024. Automated-detection of risky alcohol use prior to surgery using natural language processing. *Alcohol: Clinical and Experimental Research (Hoboken)* 48(1):153–163. https://doi.org/10.1111/acer.15222.

Wang, M., M. S. Pantell, L. M. Gottlieb, and J. Adler-Milstein. 2021. Documentation and review of social determinants of health data in the EHR: Measures and associated insights. *Journal of the American Medical Informatics Association* 28(12):2608–2616. https://doi.org/10.1093/jamia/ocab194.

WHO (World Health Organization). 2001. *International classification of functioning, disability and health: ICF.* Geneva, Switzerland: World Health Organization.

Winsor, J., J. Butterworth, A. Migliore, D. Domin, A. Zalewska, J. Shepard, E. Kamau, R. Wedeking, and J. Edelstein. 2023. *Summary of state data: The national report on employment services and outcomes through 2021.* https://www.thinkwork.org/data-note-88-summary-statedata-national-report-employment-services-and-outcomes-through-2021 (accessed June 13, 2024).

Wright, A., D. F. Sittig, J. S. Ash, D. W. Bates, J. Feblowitz, G. Fraser, S. M. Maviglia, C. McMullen, W. P. Nichol, J. E. Pang, J. Starmer, and B. Middleton. 2011. Governance for clinical decision support: Case studies and recommended practices from leading institutions. *Journal of the American Medical Informatics Association* 18(2):187–194. https://doi.org/10.1136/jamia.2009.002030.

Zuckerman, B. L., J. M. Karabin, R. A. Parker, W. E. J. Doane, and S. R. Williams. 2022. *Options and opportunities to address and mitigate the existing and potential risks, as well as promote benefits, associated with AI and other advanced analytic methods.* OPRE Report 2022-253. https://www.acf.hhs.gov/sites/default/files/documents/opre/options_and_opportunities_migitage_risks_dec2022.pdf (accessed June 13, 2024).

Appendix B

Statement of Task

A planning committee of the National Academies of Sciences, Engineering, and Medicine will plan and host a public workshop on the variety of different experiences with the U.S. healthcare system common to individuals facing barriers,[1] including members of racial or ethnic minorities, and the consequences of those different experiences on an individual's health status and medical record, which is relevant to the U.S. Social Security Administration (SSA) in disability determinations. The workshop shall include presentations with a focus on how individual's different experiences can manifest in records, as well as medical advances, developments, and research related to health inequities in the United States.

The workshop will feature invited presentations and panel discussions on topics such as:

- The primary social determinants of health affecting people facing barriers and members of racial or ethnic minorities, how they might be reflected in medical records, and how they differ between and among various groups.
- Societal, systemic, racial, cultural, or personal characteristics that can serve as impediments to people facing barriers and members of racial or ethnic minorities seeking or receiving medical services and, in particular:

---

[1] Including people with low income, limited English proficiency, facing homelessness, or with mental illness.

    a. How those characteristics may be recorded or manifest in traditional and other healthcare records;

    b. How the medical records of people with those characteristics might differ from the general population; and

    c. How the impact of those impediments can be lessened or averted, particularly in the context of consultative examinations ordered by SSA.

- The lived experiences of people facing barriers and members of racial or ethnic minorities as they interact with SSA, healthcare systems, and alternative sources of medical care, including:

    a. How those experiences impact future use of or trust in medical or healthcare services;

    b. Disconnects between the health-related reports made by people facing barriers and the information recorded by their healthcare providers;

    c. Are there alternative sources of medical care utilized by some people facing barriers; and

    d. Areas of difficulty or confusion when making a disability application, providing SSA with medical and other records, or attending a consultative examination.

- An overview of recent or emerging research suggesting particular widely-used tests or procedures are not as accurate or appropriate as traditionally believed for certain sub-populations and, for each, whether alternate tests or procedures exist which have been found to be accurate and appropriate for the population in question.

The planning committee shall develop the agenda for the workshop sessions, select and invite speakers and discussants, and moderate the discussions. The speakers and discussants will have the experience and knowledge to speak to the differences experienced by various racial and ethnic populations and other groups of people facing barriers. A proceedings of the presentations and discussions at the workshop will be prepared by a designated rapporteur in accordance with institutional guidelines.

Appendix C

Workshop Agenda

9:00 AM **Welcome and Goals for the Workshop Day 1**
- **Amy J. Houtrow,** Planning Committee Cochair
- **Karrie A. Shogren,** Planning Committee Cochair

9:10 AM **Sponsor Opening Remarks**
- **Michael Goldstein,** U.S. Social Security Administration

9:15 AM **SESSION I: OVERVIEW, CONCEPTS, AND FRAMING**
Moderator: Karrie A. Shogren, Planning Committee Cochair

Definition of Disability
- **Amy J. Houtrow,** Planning Committee Cochair

SSA Disability Determinations Process Overview
- **Vincent Nibali,** U.S. Social Security Administration

Basics of Health Disparities
- **Jonathan Platt,** Planning Committee Member

The Purpose and Function of the Medical Record
- **Kensaku Kawamoto,** Planning Committee Member

9:55 AM   **SESSION II: SOCIAL DETERMINANTS OF HEALTH AND THEIR EFFECT ON CARE**
Moderator: **Ruqaiijah Yearby,** Planning Committee Member

Panelist Remarks
- **Monika Mitra,** Brandeis University
- **Joy Amaryllis Johnson,** Charlottesville Public Housing Association of Residents, and Disability Advocate
- **Benjamin F. Miller,** Stanford School of Medicine
- **Jennifer Hudson,** Williamson Health and Wellness Center

Q&A with the Panelists

11:00 AM   **BREAK**

11:15 AM   **SESSION III: DISPARITIES AND BIAS IN EVALUATIVE TESTING AND RECORDING OF MEDICAL INFORMATION**
Rupa Valdez, Planning Committee Member

Panelist Remarks
- **Marshall H. Chin,** University of Chicago
- **Gloria Thornton,** Amplified Disabled Voices, and Disability Advocate
- **Tara Lagu,** Northwestern University Feinberg School of Medicine
- **AJ Link,** Autistic Self Advocacy Network, and Disability Advocate

Q&A with the Panelists

12:30 PM   **BREAK FOR LUNCH**

1:30 PM   **SESSION IV: HEALTH DISPARITIES AND THE DISABILITY APPLICATION PROCESS**
Moderator: **Amanda Alise Price,** Planning Committee Member

Panelist Remarks
- **Bonnielin Swenor,** Johns Hopkins Medicine
- **D'Sena' Warren,** Disability Advocate
- **Yvonne M. Perret,** Advocacy and Training Center

Q&A with the Panelists

2:45 PM   **BREAK**

3:00 PM   **SESSION V: MITIGATING THE EFFECT OF
              HEALTH DISPARITIES IN THE SSA DISABILITY
              DETERMINATION PROCESS**
              Moderator: **Michael V. Stanton,** Planning Committee Member

              Panel discussion will include selected speakers from previous
              sessions.
              • **Marshall H. Chin,** University of Chicago
              • **Yvonne M. Perret,** Advocacy and Training Center
              • **D'Sena' Warren,** Disability Advocate
              • **Monika Mitra,** Brandeis University

3:45 PM   **Closing Reflections**
              • **Amy J. Houtrow,** Planning Committee Cochair
              • **Karrie A. Shogren,** Planning Committee Cochair

4:00 PM   **ADJOURN DAY 1**

              APRIL 5, 2024: 9:00 AM – 2:30 PM EDT

9:00 AM   **Welcome and Goals for the Workshop Day 2**
              • **Karrie A. Shogren,** Planning Committee Cochair

9:10 AM   **Day 1 Recap**
              • **Amy J. Houtrow,** Planning Committee Cochair

9:20 AM   **SESSION VI: THE HEALTH RECORD IN DEPTH**
              Moderator: **Kensaku Kawamoto,** Planning Committee Member

              Panelist Remarks
              • **S. Trent Rosenbloom,** Vanderbilt University Medical Center
              • **Guilherme Del Fiol,** University of Utah Medical School
              • **Julia Adler-Milstein,** University of California San Francisco
              • **V.G. Vinod Vydiswaran,** University of Michigan

              Q&A with the Panelists

10:30 AM   **BREAK**

10:45 AM   **SESSION VII: THE RELATIONSHIP BETWEEN THE
            MEDICAL RECORD AND HEALTH DISPARITIES**
            Moderator: **Kenrick Cato,** Planning Committee Member

            Panelist Remarks
            • **Megan Morris,** University of Colorado Anschutz Medical
              Center
            • **Carolyn Petersen,** Mayo Clinic
            • **Prerana Laddha,** Epic Systems
            • **Julia Skapik,** National Association of Community Health
              Centers

            Q&A with the Panelists

12:00 PM   **BREAK FOR LUNCH**

1:00 PM   **SESSION VIII: APPROACHES TO ADVANCING
            MEDICAL RECORDS TO ADDRESS DISPARITIES IN
            DISABILITY DETERMINATIONS**
            Moderator: **Elham Mahmoudi,** Planning Committee Member

            Panel discussion will include selected speakers from previous
            sessions.
            • **Megan Morris,** University of Colorado Anschutz Medical
              Center
            • **Julia Adler-Milstein,** University of California San Francisco
            • **Bonnielin Swenor,** Johns Hopkins Medicine
            • **V.G. Vinod Vydiswaran,** University of Michigan
            • **D'Sena' Warren,** Disability Advocate
            • **Prerana Laddha,** Epic Systems
            • **Tara Lagu,** Northwestern University Feinberg School of
              Medicine

2:15 PM   **Closing Reflections**
            • **Amy J. Houtrow,** Planning Committee Cochair
            • **Karrie A. Shogren,** Planning Committee Cochair

2:30 PM   **ADJOURN DAY 2**

Appendix D

Biographical Sketches of Planning Committee Members and Speakers

PLANNING COMMITTEE

AMY J. HOUTROW, M.D., Ph.D., M.P.H. (Cochair), is a professor and Vice Chair in the Department of Physical Medicine and Rehabilitation for Pediatric Rehabilitation Medicine at the University of Pittsburgh School of Medicine. She is also the Vice Chair for Quality and Outcomes. She is the Chief of Pediatric Rehabilitation Medicine Services at the University of Pittsburgh Medical Center's Children's Hospital of Pittsburgh. Complementing her clinical focus, Dr. Houtrow's research focus is recognizing the effects that raising children with disabilities has on families and developing channels to improve service delivery. She works closely with leaders in health services research around the country. Dr. Houtrow is a collaborator on the DIVERSE Collective that is investigating health equity as it relates to children with disabilities.

KARRIE A. SHOGREN, Ph.D. (Cochair), is the director of the Kansas University Center on Developmental Disabilities (a University Center for Excellence in Developmental Disabilities), senior scientist at the Schiefelbusch Life Span Institute, and Ross and Marianna Beach Distinguished Professor in the Department of Special Education, all at the University of Kansas. Dr. Shogren's research focuses on assessment and intervention in self-determination and supported decision making for people with disabilities. Dr. Shogren has led multiple grant-funded projects, including assessment validation and efficacy trials of self-determination interventions in school and community contexts. Dr. Shogren has published more than 225 articles in peer-reviewed journals, is the author or coauthor of 25 books, and is the lead author of the Self-Determination Inventory, a recently validated assessment of self-determination and the Supported Decision-Making Inventory System, an assessment of the supports needed to involve people with intellectual and developmental disabilities in decisions about their lives. Dr. Shogren has received grant funding from several sources, including the Institute of Education Sciences and the National Institute on Disability, Independent Living, and Rehabilitation Research. Dr. Shogren is coeditor of *Remedial and Special Education* and a Fellow of the American Association on Intellectual and Developmental Disabilities and the American Psychological Association.

KENRICK CATO, Ph.D., RN, CPHIMS, FAAN, is a clinical informatician whose research focuses on mining electronic patient data to support decision making for clinicians, patients, and caregivers. Operationally, he spends his time mining and modeling nursing data to optimize nursing value in health care. He is also involved in several national-level informatics organizations, including as a board member of the American Medical Informatics Association (AMIA), Chair of the Nursing Informatics Working Group (NIWG) of AMIA, as well as a convening member of the AMIA-sponsored 25 x 5 initiative to reduce documentation burden. Dr. Cato received his B.S.N., M.S., and Ph.D. in clinical informatics at Columbia University.

KENSAKU KAWAMOTO, M.D., Ph.D., M.H.S., FACMI, FAMIA, is a professor of biomedical informatics and the Associate Chief Medical Information Officer at the University of Utah. He is also the founding director of ReImagine EHR, a multistakeholder initiative to improve patient care and the provider experience through interoperable electronic health record (EHR) innovations that convert data to actionable insight. An expert on the practical and scalable use of digital technologies to improve health and health care, Dr. Kawamoto cochairs the Clinical Decision Support (CDS) Work Group of HL7, the primary standards development organization for health IT. He also served as co-initiative coordinator for the Clinical Quality Framework (CQF), a public–private partnership sponsored by the Office of the National Coordinator for Health Information Technology and the Centers for Medicare & Medicaid Services that developed and validated a harmonized set of standards for CDS and electronic clinical quality measurement. He also served two terms on the U.S. Health IT Advisory Committee. Dr. Kawamoto is a fellow of the American College of Medical Informatics and was recognized by *Modern Healthcare* as a Top Innovator. His formal training includes a B.A. in Biochemical Sciences from Harvard and an M.D., a Ph.D. in Biomedical Engineering, and an M.H.S. in Clinical Research from Duke University.

ELHAM MAHMOUDI, Ph.D., is an associate professor of health economics at the University of Michigan Department of Family Medicine. She is a mixed methods researcher, with expertise in using administrative claims data. Her research focuses on evaluating health care policies aimed at reducing racial and ethnic disparities in access to care and quality of care, and it extends to examining health care use, cost, and efficiency of care for older adults with Alzheimer's disease and related dementias.

JONATHAN PLATT, Ph.D., M.P.H., is a social and psychiatric epidemiologist whose research focuses on the identification of social causes of suicide, psychiatric disorders, and harmful substance use in order to identify key targets to improve public health and reduce group disparities. He has expertise in the measurement of social structures, causal inference methods, and longitudinal data analysis to identify the health consequences of social inequities across the life course. He also has growing expertise in the use of machine learning methods to identify novel health risk patterns and satisfy causal inference assumptions. Dr. Platt has published more than 40 articles and book chapters (h-index: 24), in leading public health and psychiatry journals, including the *New England Journal of Medicine*, *JAMA Psychiatry*, *American Journal of Epidemiology*, and *Social Science & Medicine*. He is an active member in the broader public health research community, participating in major conferences in the fields of population science, epidemiologic methods, and psychiatry and serves as an ad hoc reviewer for numerous journals and as a review editor for the journal *Frontiers in Global Women's Health*. He is an early-stage academic researcher (tenure track) in the department of epidemiology at the University of Iowa College of Public Health.

AMANDA ALISE PRICE, Ph.D., became the director of the Office of Health Equity as well as the *Eunice Kennedy Shriver* National Institute of Child Health and Human Development (NICHD) chief scientific diversity officer in April 2023. In these roles, she leads the effort to shape the institute's vision for diversity, equity, inclusion, and accessibility. As part of her duties, she leads NICHD's STrategies to enRich Inclusion and achieVe Equity (STRIVE) Initiative, guiding it into implementation following finalization of the STRIVE Action Plan. She also provides guidance and serves as a technical authority on health disparities and health equity research across NICHD's extramural and intramural programs. Dr. Price joined NIH in 2020 as a health scientist administrator and program director. She most recently directed the preventive medicine portfolio and served as a team lead of the Division of Extramural Science Programs at the National Institute of Nursing Research. She previously worked at the National Cancer Institute's Center for Reducing Cancer Health Disparities. Throughout her NIH career, she has served on several

NIH-wide committees and coauthored concepts and funding opportunities to stimulate health disparity and health equity research, increase inclusion for underrepresented populations in research, and promote scientific workforce diversity. Prior to joining NIH, Dr. Price was a tenured associate professor in the School of Health Sciences at Winston-Salem State University, a minority-serving institution that is designated as a Historically Black College and University. She taught, trained, and mentored underrepresented scholars in research and the biomedical sciences. She also successfully competed for NIH funding as a principal investigator and generated publications and presentations from her work, which centered on preventing and managing chronic diseases through promotion of healthy lifestyle behaviors, with an emphasis on addressing health disparities and promoting health equity. Dr. Price earned both a Ph.D. and B.S.Ed. in exercise physiology, with a doctoral concentration in statistics, and undergraduate minors in chemistry and sports medicine from the University of Miami in Coral Gables, Florida.

MICHAEL V. STANTON, Ph.D., is a licensed clinical health psychologist and associate professor of public health at California State University, East Bay, a diverse minority-serving institution in Northern California. Dr. Stanton's research has been cited over 3,700 times and examines how stress, including discrimination and stigma, affects health, with a particular focus on eating behavior. His clinical work integrates mindfulness with cognitive behavioral therapy to treat mental and physical health concerns. Dr. Stanton has held multiple leadership positions, including at the Society of Behavioral Medicine and the American Psychosomatic Society, and he currently serves on its Leadership Council. He contributes his expertise to the field as a Consulting Editor and Editorial Fellow at the *American Psychological Association Journal, Health Psychology*, and to the general public as a guest contributor to several news stations, including ABC, NBC, CBS, NPR, the *San Francisco Chronicle,* and other media, where he adds psychology and public health expertise to the analysis of current events. He is a former NHLBI-sponsored UCSF-RISE Fellow and Fulbright Fellow. He earned his Ph.D. in clinical psychology with a focus in behavioral medicine from Duke University, completed his post-doctoral training at Stanford University School of Medicine, and received his B.A. from Brown University.

RUPA VALDEZ, Ph.D., is an associate professor at the University of Virginia with joint appointments in the School of Engineering and Applied Sciences and the School of Medicine and serves as president of the Blue Trunk Foundation. Dr. Valdez merges the disciplines of human factors engineering, health informatics, and cultural anthropology to understand and support the ways in which people manage health at home and in the community. Her work draws heavily on community engagement with community organizations and individuals from multiple health disparity populations, and has been supported by the NIH, AHRQ, NSF, and USDA, among others. She has testified before Congress on the topic of health equity for the disability community and received the Jack A. Kraft Innovator Award from the Human Factors and Ergonomics Society (HFES). Among other appointments, she serves as associate editor for the *Journal of American Medical Informatics Association Open*, on the Board of Directors for the American Association of People with Disabilities, and as an advisor for PCORI's Patient Engagement Advisory Panel and for NCQA's Health Equity Expert Work Group. Dr. Valdez received her Ph.D. at the University of Wisconsin-Madison.

RUQAIIJAH YEARBY, J.D., M.P.H., is the inaugural Kara J. Trott Professor in Health Law at the Moritz College of Law, professor in the department of health services management and policy at the College of Public Health, and a faculty affiliate of the Kirwan Institute for the Study of Race and Ethnicity at the Ohio State University. An expert in health policy and civil rights, Professor Yearby has received over $5 million from the National Institutes of Health (NIH) to study structural racism and discrimination in vaccine allocation and from the Robert Wood Johnson Foundation to study the equitable enforcement of housing laws and structural racism in the health care system. She was one of the keynote speakers for the 5th Annual Conference of the ELSI Congress and has served as a reviewer for NIH, the Swiss National Science Foundation, and the Wellcome Trust. She is on the editorial board of the *American Journal of Bioethics*. She is a Committee Member for the U.S. Department of Health and Human Services, Secretary's Advisory Committee on Human Research Protections. Her work has been published in the *American Journal of Bioethics*, *American Journal of Public Health*, *Health Affairs*, and the *Oxford Journal of Law and the Biosciences*.

SPEAKER BIOSKETCHES

JULIA ADLER-MILSTEIN, Ph.D., is a professor of medicine, chief of the Division of Clinical Informatics & Digital Transformation, and Director of the Center for Clinical Informatics & Improvement Research (CLIIR). Dr. Adler-Milstein is a leading researcher in health IT policy, with a specific focus on electronic health records and interoperability. She has examined policies and organizational strategies that enable effective use of electronic health records and promote interoperability. She is also an expert in EHR audit log data and its application to studying clinician behavior. Her research—used by researchers, health systems, and policy makers—identifies obstacles to progress and ways to overcome them.

She has published more than 200 influential papers, testified before the U.S. Senate Health, Education, Labor and Pensions Committee, is a member of the National Academy of Medicine, been named one of the top 10 influential women in health IT, and won numerous awards, including the New Investigator Award from the American Medical Informatics Association and the Alice S. Hersh New Investigator Award from AcademyHealth. She has served on an array of influential committees and boards, including the NHS National Advisory Group on Health Information Technology, the Health Care Advisory Board for *Politico*, and the Interoperability Committee of the National Quality Forum. Dr. Adler-Milstein holds a Ph.D. in health policy from Harvard and spent 6 years on the faculty at University of Michigan prior to joining UCSF as a professor in the Department of Medicine and the inaugural director of the Center for Clinical Informatics and Improvement Research in 2017. She became the inaugural chief of the Division of Clinical Informatics and Digital Transformation in 2023.

MARSHALL H. CHIN, M.D., M.P.H., Richard Parrillo Family Distinguished Service Professor of Healthcare Ethics at the University of Chicago, is a practicing general internist and health services researcher who has dedicated his career to advancing health equity through interventions at individual, organizational, community, and policy levels. Through the Robert Wood Johnson Foundation Advancing Health Equity: Leading Care, Payment, and Systems Transformation program, Dr. Chin collaborates with teams of state Medicaid agencies, Medicaid managed care organizations, frontline health care delivery organizations, and community-based organizations to implement payment reforms to support and incentivize care transformations that advance health equity within an antiracist framework. He also cochairs the Centers for Medicare & Medicaid Services Health Care Payment Learning and Action Network Health Equity Advisory Team.

Dr. Chin evaluates the value of the federally qualified health center program, improves diabetes outcomes in Chicago's South Side through health care and community interventions, and improves shared decision making among clinicians and LGBTQ persons of color. He also applies ethical principles to reforms to advance health equity, discussions about a culture of equity, and what it means for health professionals to care and advocate for their patients. Dr. Chin uses improv and standup comedy, storytelling, and theater to improve the training of students in caring for diverse patients and engaging in constructive discussions around systemic racism and social privilege. Dr. Chin is a graduate of Harvard College and the University of California at San Francisco School of Medicine, and he completed residency and fellowship training in general internal medicine at Brigham and Women's Hospital, Harvard Medical School. He has received mentoring awards from the Society of General Internal Medicine and the University of Chicago. He is a former President of the Society of General Internal Medicine. Dr. Chin was elected to the National Academy of Medicine in 2017 and is on the Steering Committee for the NAM paper series on structural racism and health.

GUILHERME DEL FIOL, M.S., M.D. Ph.D., earned his M.D. from the University of Sao Paulo, Brazil; his M.S. in information systems from the Catholic University of Parana, Brazil; and his Ph.D. in biomedical informatics from the University of Utah. He is currently professor and vice chair for research in the University of Utah's Department of Biomedical Informatics. Prior to the University of Utah, Dr. Del Fiol held positions in clinical knowl-edge management at Intermountain Healthcare and as faculty at the Duke Community and Family Medicine Department. Since 2008, he has served as an elected cochair of the Clinical Decision Support Work Group at Health Level International (HL7). He is also an elected fellow of the American College of Medical Informatics (ACMI) and a member of the Comprehensive Cancer Center at Huntsman Cancer Institute.

Dr. Del Fiol's research interests are in the design, development, evaluation, and dissemination of standards-based clinical decision support and digital health interventions. He has been focusing particularly on interventions to improve cancer prevention and reduce health disparities. He is the lead author of the HL7 Infobutton Standard and the project lead for OpenInfobutton, an open source suite of infobutton tools and Web services, which is in production use at several health care organizations throughout the United States, including Intermountain Healthcare, Duke University, and the Veterans Health Administration (VHA). His research has been funded by various sources, including the National Library of Medicine (NLM), National Cancer Institute (NCI), Agency for Healthcare Research and Quality, Centers for Disease Control and Prevention, Centers for Medicare and Medicaid Services, and Patient-Centered Outcomes Research Institute.

JENNIFER HUDSON is development director for a federally qualified health center in southern West Virginia. She brings together resources behind efforts including the reopening of a rural hospital and growing a commercial kitchen and clothing store. She believes in systems of care that invest in building community infrastructure and support to serve individuals and their families.

JOY AMARYLLIS JOHNSON currently works for the Charlottesville Redevelopment and Housing Authority as its resident services/Section 3 coordinator. She helps connect residents with a variety of resources and work with contractors to set up interviews with residents. She previously worked as an Outreach Coordinator for the Westhaven Nursing Clinic in Charlottesville,

Virginia, for more than 20 years. Ms. Johnson has been a longtime community activist and organizer working to address low-income housing issues at the local and national levels. She has volunteered countless hours as an advocate for Charlottesville's low-income residents, speaking out on their behalf to demand safe and clean affordable housing, adequate representation on city boards and commissions, living wage employment, and voter education. In 1998, Ms. Johnson helped found the Public Housing Association of Residents (PHAR), a nationally recognized citywide resident association, which is responsible for the city's outstanding level of resident representation on its Housing Authority Board of Commissioners.

She is a former member of the Charlottesville Redevelopment and Housing Authority Board of Commissioners. She also previously served on the Head Start Policy Council, University of Virginia Employee Council, Virginia Association of Neighborhoods, Offender Aid and Restoration Board, Westhaven Tenant Association, Everywhere and Now Public Housing Residents Organizing Nationally Together (ENPHRONT), National Low Income Housing Coalition (NLIHC), Monticello Area Community Action Agency (MACAA), Connecting People to Jobs, Charlottesville CBDG Task Force, Charlottesville Housing Advisory Committee, and Charlottesville Social Services Advisory Board.

Currently, Ms. Johnson serves as Chair for the Public Housing Association of Residents (PHAR), Vice President of the Board of Legal Aid Justice Center, Chair for Charlottesville Housing Advisory Committee, and UVA Housing Committee.

Ms. Johnson received training with a certificate from Nan McKay as a Public Housing Specialist. She has also received training with HUD on Public Housing Assessment Scores, Section 3, Train the Trainer I and II as well as with the National Low Income Housing Coalition on the Quality Housing and Work Responsibility Act and Section 3. She has also received training and attended workshops with LAOSHAC, the Babcock Foundation, and the Legal Aid Justice Center. She is the recipient of the 2020 Cushing Niles Dolbeare lifetime service award and 2023 Reflector Award.

PRERANA LADDHA serves as the director of Social Care and Behavioral Health at Epic Systems. In this role, she leads global product development in the areas of continuing care and population health. With over a decade of experience in health care and a master's degree in computer science, she is driven by a commitment to using technology and research to foster the well-being of individuals and communities across the globe.

Laddha was instrumental in leading Epic's development projects to advance the integration of social drivers of health into electronic medical records, connect patients with community resources, and close loops on community referrals. Prerana's influence extends beyond national boundaries; she has collaborated with Finland, Norway, Northern Ireland, and Australia to deeply understand and address social needs on a global scale. Notably, she led the development project to implement the world's first integrated health and social record in Finland. She has represented Epic at the White House and is part of the White House Challenge to end hunger and build healthy communities across the nation. Additionally, as a member of the Alignment of Progress, she advises on national strategies for mental health and substance abuse disorders, aiming to inform policy makers and advocate for standardized, measurement-based care.

Her global experience has equipped her with valuable insights, which she uses to guide Epic's client community toward best practices in governance, implementation, interoperability, and outcome measurement within social and behavioral health workflows. Her blend of computer science expertise and a passionate commitment to social and behavioral health challenges empowers her to champion innovative technology solutions that address complex social and mental health issues.

TARA LAGU, M.D., M.P.H., is professor of medicine and medical social sciences and the Director of the Center for Health Services and Outcomes Research in the Institute for Public Health and Medicine at Northwestern University Feinberg School of Medicine. She is a pharmacist, hospitalist, and health services researcher with expertise in application of mixed methods to measure quality of health care, observational comparative effectiveness, and implementation science. She is passionate about influencing policy and improving care for vulnerable and marginalized patients, including patients with heart failure (HF) and disability. After completing a degree in pharmacy from Purdue University, an M.D./M.P.H. at the Yale University School of Medicine, and a General Internal Medicine Residency at Rhode Island Hospital/Warren Alpert Medical School/Brown University, Dr. Lagu was a Robert Wood Johnson Clinical Scholar at the University of Pennsylvania from 2005 to 2008. She has published about 150 original peer-reviewed manuscripts in high-impact journals, including the *New England Journal of Medicine* (*NEJM*), *JAMA*, the *Annals of Internal Medicine*, and *Health Affairs*.

In 2013, Dr. Lagu was inspired by her clinical work as a hospitalist to focus a portion of her research on gaps in access to care for patients with disabilities. Using a "secret shopper" approach, she found that 20 percent of outpatient physicians nationwide would refuse to see a patient who uses a wheelchair. In 2022, Dr. Lagu, with senior author Dr. Lisa Iezzoni, led on a study that showed that physicians make strategic decisions to refuse to care for patients with disabilities. This work was published in *Health Affairs*, profiled in the *New York Times*, and featured on NPR's "Science Friday." Dr. Lagu is using this work to launch efforts to improve care delivery for patients with disabilities and to rethink and redesign medical education around people with disabilities. Dr. Lagu also serves as a standing member of the NIH Health Services: Quality and Effectiveness study section and on the editorial board for the *Journal of Hospital Medicine.* She was the winner of the 2019 Society of Hospital Medicine Award for Excellence in Research and was named one of the American College of Physicians "Top Hospitalists" in 2019.

AJ LINK, J.D. LL.M., is openly autistic. He received his J.D. from the George Washington University Law School and his LL.M in space law at the University of Mississippi School of Law. He is the inaugural director of the Center for Air and Space Law Task Force on Inclusion, Diversity, and Equity in Aerospace and an adjunct professor of space law at Howard University School of Law. Link works as a research director for the Jus Ad Astra project and previously served as the Communications Director for AstroAccess. He is the Space Law and Policy Chair for Black in Astro and was the founding president of the National Disabled Law Students Association. He also helped found the National Disabled Legal Professionals Association and is a commissioner on the American Bar Association Commission on Disability Rights.

He is a policy analyst for the Autistic Self Advocacy Network. He has been actively involved with disability advocacy in the Washington, DC, area and nationally within the United States. He serves on several advisory boards and steering committees that focus on disability advocacy and broader social justice movements.

BENJAMIN F. MILLER, Psy.D., a clinical psychologist by training, is an academic, executive, and policy expert. Over the last 2 decades, Dr. Miller has worked to prioritize mental health in policies, programs, and investments. He works at the intersection of policy and practice, ensuring that mental health and substance misuse solutions are a focus across the world.

Dr. Miller's expertise in the mental health space largely stems from the early days of his career. Beginning as an educator, teaching special education, he saw firsthand how systems fail those who are in the most need. After receiving his doctorate in clinical psychology from Spalding University in Louisville, he began his years-long professional relationship with the University of Colorado School of Medicine, beginning with his predoctoral internship at Colorado in 2006. He subsequently trained at the University of Massachusetts Medical School, focusing on how to better integrate mental health into primary care.

After returning to Colorado from Massachusetts, he joined the Department of Family Medicine, where he worked for more than 8 years, ultimately achieving the academic rank of Associate Professor. During his tenure at

Colorado, he helped establish the Eugene S. Farley, Jr., Health Policy Center as its founding director. The Farley Center positioned Miller as a national thought leader on mental health and policy and led to the creation of several seminal documents and publications. From Colorado, he transitioned to help start Well Being Trust, a national foundation that focused on advancing the mental, social, and spiritual health of the nation. Under his leadership as president of the foundation, Well Being Trust helped invest in the creation of several movement-building organizations, reports that influenced policy change, and tools that could be used by communities to advance mental health.

With more than 100 publications and hundreds of invited keynote speaking engagements, Miller has fought relentlessly to change the national narrative around mental health.

MONIKA MITRA, Ph.D., is the Nancy Lurie Marks Professor of Disability Policy and director of the Lurie Institute for Disability Policy at Brandeis University. Her research broadly focuses on disparities in health outcomes and health care access among people with disabilities. She leads several federally funded projects, including the National Research Center for Parents with Disabilities, which is focused on addressing knowledge gaps regarding the needs of parents with diverse disabilities and their families, and the Community Living Policy Center, which is aimed at improving policies and practices that advance community living outcomes for people with disabilities. Dr. Mitra is also the co-PI of the recently launched Center for Disability and Pregnancy Research and is co-Editor-in-Chief of the *Disability and Health Journal.*

MEGAN MORRIS, Ph.D., M.P.H., CCC-SLP, is an associate professor in the Division of General Internal Medicine at the University of Colorado Anschutz Medical Campus. Her research aims to identify and address the multilevel conditions that contribute to the provision of equitable care for people with disabilities. She is a leading expert on the documentation of patients' disability status in the electronic health record and health care disparities experienced by patients with communication disabilities. Dr. Morris is the founder and director of the Disability Equity Collaborative, a community aimed at advancing equitable care for patients with disabilities through practice, policy, and research. Dr. Morris's research and advocacy has been shaped by both her personal and professional experiences of ableism in the health care setting.

YVONNE M. PERRET, M.A., M.S.W., LCSW-C, is a psychiatric clinical social worker with more than 45 years of experience. She is the executive director of the Advocacy and Training Center in Cumberland, Maryland, and has a master's degree in journalism. She is the coauthor of a book on children with disabilities (three editions) as well as two book chapters and several articles on SSI/SSDI and related mental health topics. She has written curricula on mental illness, homelessness, and recovery; on co-occurring disorders; on self-compassion; on identifying and working with shelter residents' strengths; and on brain injury and homelessness for the New York State Office of Temporary Disability Assistance. She trains these curricula to NYC and NYS shelter and Department of Social Services staff.

Ms. Perret is the primary founder of SOAR (SSI/SSDI Outreach, Access and Recovery), a national program that includes a SOAR TA Center based in Albany, New York, which is funded by Substance Abuse and Mental Health Services Administration (SAMHSA). SOAR focuses on assisting adults who are homeless with accessing SSI/SSDI in an expedited way and beginning their recovery both from homelessness and mental illness and/or co-occurring disorders. In 2001, the Baltimore SSI Outreach Project, the program on which SOAR is based and which Ms. Perret directed, was named a Best Practice Program by the National Alliance to End Homelessness and, in 2005, an Exemplary Practice Program by SAMHSA. As part of SOAR, she is the lead author of Stepping Stones to Recovery (funded by SAMHSA) and Stepping Stones to SSI/SSDI (funded by HUD HOPWA), two curricula that focus on assisting individuals with accessing SSI/SSDI and beginning recovery. The emphasis in both curricula is on using benefits as tools in recovery. Ms. Perret has worked in 47 states promoting SOAR and working with community teams, including SSA and DDS, to promote collaboration, training, and planning.

Ms. Perret has also trained and worked extensively in co-occurring disorders, mental illness, and other mental health-related topics. She has presented at numerous mental health and other national conferences and is the recipient of several awards for mental health advocacy. Most recently, she was named one of Maryland's Top 100 Women by the *Daily Record*, the Maryland publication for government, business, and legal news.

CAROLYN PETERSEN, M.S., M.B.I., FAMIA, is an assistant professor in the Department of Artificial Intelligence and Informatics at Mayo Clinic and senior editor of the consumer health information website MayoClinic.org. She holds a Master of Science in Exercise and Movement Science from the University of Oregon and a Master of Biomedical Informatics from Oregon Health & Science University. She previously cochaired the Health Information Technology Advisory Committee for the Office of the National Coordinator for Health Information Technology and has served on FDA medical device advisory panels and the Patient-Centered Outcomes Research Institute's Advisory Panel on Healthcare Delivery and Disparities Research. A long-term pediatric cancer survivor, Ms. Petersen's work focuses on patient engagement and experience, person-generated health data and data governance, health equity, and ethics and technology.

S. TRENT ROSENBLOOM, M.D., M.P.H., FACMI, FAAP, FAMIA, is the vice chair for faculty affairs and a professor of biomedical informatics with secondary appointments in medicine, pediatrics, and the School of Nursing at Vanderbilt University. He is a board-certified Internist and Pediatrician who earned his M.D., completed a residency in Internal Medicine and Pediatrics, a fellowship in Biomedical Informatics, and earned an M.P.H. all at Vanderbilt. Dr. Rosenbloom is a nationally recognized investigator in the field of health information technology evaluation. His research has focused on studying how health care providers, patients, and caregivers interact with health information technologies when documenting medical and health-related activities, and when making clinical decisions. Dr. Rosenbloom is the director for My Health at Vanderbilt, one of the nation's oldest and best adopted patient portals that now has over one million users.

Dr. Rosenbloom has successfully competed for extramural funding from the National Library of Medicine, the Agency for Healthcare Research and Quality, and the Patient-Centered Outcomes Research Institute. Dr. Rosenbloom's work has resulted in lead and collaborating authorship on over 100 peer-reviewed manuscripts, which have been published in the *Journal of the American Medical Informatics Association*, *Pediatrics*, *Annals of Internal Medicine*, and *Academic Medicine*, among others. In addition, Dr. Rosenbloom has authored and coauthored six book chapters and numerous posters, white papers and invited papers. He has been a committed member of the principal professional organization in his field, the American Medical Informatics Association (AMIA). He has served AMIA in leadership roles, including participating in the Board of Directors, the Journal and Publications Committee, Scientific Program Committees, the *Journal of the American Medical Informatics Association* (JAMIA) Editorial Board, several national Health Policy Meetings, the JAMIA Editor-in-Chief search committee, and a Working Group on Unintended Consequences. As a result of his research success and service to AMIA, Dr. Rosenbloom was the annual recipient of the competitive AMIA New Investigator Award in 2009, was elected to the American College of Medical Informatics (ACMI) in 2011 and as a Fellow of the American Medical Informatics Association (FAMIA) in 2020, and granted an AMIA Leadership Award in 2023. In addition, Dr. Rosenbloom has participated in study sections for the National Library of Medicine, the Agency for Healthcare Research and Quality in Healthcare, the National Science Foundation, and the Patient-Centered Outcomes Research Institute.

Dr. Rosenbloom has participated as a mentor for numerous students, including Ph.D. candidates from Biomedical Informatics and medical students performing research projects. He has been an advisor to medical students and is a faculty affiliate advisor for the School of Medicine's Chapman Advisory College. He is an associate director for the Vanderbilt Medical Innovators Development Program (MIDP), a 4-year M.D. training program tailored to engineers and applied scientists that teaches them to solve clinical problems by translating discoveries in engineering into valuable innovations.

JULIA SKAPIK, M.D., M.P.H., is the medical director for informatics at National Association of Community Health Centers (NACHC) and a board-certified Internist and Clinical Informaticist. She came to NACHC after a stint as the Chief Health Information Officer for Cognitive Medical Systems after 5 years as a Senior Medical Informatics Officer at ONC. Dr. Skapik is also an ongoing leader in HIT interoperability, governance, and clinical content as the Chief Medical Informatics Officer for Logica Health and in standards development as a member of the HL7 Board of Directors. In her role at NACHC, Dr. Skapik is focused on broad HIT stakeholder coordination and engagement, common data definitions and measure harmonization, and HIT-enabled clinical quality improvement, care coordination, and patient engagement.

BONNIELIN SWENOR, Ph.D., M.P.H., is an epidemiologist and the Endowed Professor of Disability Health and Justice at The Johns Hopkins School of Nursing, with joint appointments at the Johns Hopkins School of Medicine and the Johns Hopkins Bloomberg School of Public Health. She is the founder and director of the Johns Hopkins Disability Health Research Center, which uses data-driven approaches to shift the paradigm from "living with a disability" to "thriving with a disability." Motivated by her personal experience with disability, her work is focused on advancing equity for people with disabilities, promoting disability inclusion and accessibility, and developing evidence-based and disability-inclusive policies. Dr. Swenor has provided advice and expertise to multiple organizations and agencies, including speaking at the White House Office of Science and Technology Policy (OSTP) Summit on Equity and Excellence in STEMM; chairing the National Academies of Science, Engineering, and Medicine planning committee for the Disrupting Ableism and Advancing STEM series; cochairing the NIH Advisory Committee to the Director (ACD) Subgroup on Individuals with Disabilities; and serving as a member of the Centers for Disease Control and Prevention (CDC) ACD Health Equity Workgroup. Her work has been published in leading academic journals, such as the *New England Journal of Medicine*, the *Journal of the American Medical Association*, and the *Lancet*, and has been featured in multiple news outlets, including the *New York Times*, the *Washington Post*, and *TIME* magazine. Dr. Swenor has a track record of translating research into policy change, as she played a pivotal role in national advocacy that led the NIH to designate people with disabilities as a health disparity population and recently co-led efforts outlining limitations with proposed changes to the U.S. Census Bureau disability questions.

GLORIA THORNTON, founder of Amplified Disabled Voices LLC, is an ombudsman deeply committed to disability advocacy. As a person with disabilities Gloria is well versed on medical discrepancies fueled by personal and professional drive. Gloria Thornton obtained a master's degree in human services and a bachelor's in psychology. She is currently working toward obtaining her Doctor of Human Services with a specialty in Prevention, Intervention, and Advocacy.

As a woman and a minority, she has had an abundance of lived experience that consists of barriers directly related to cultural incompetence thus resulting in medical discrepancies. Once finding a doctor who listened, she received multiple different health diagnoses that sparked the love for advocacy. When she is not advocating for herself or others, Gloria enjoys watching movies with friends, spending time with her family and dog, reading, and Dancing as a Lil Sis for the Rollettes, a Los Angeles–based wheelchair dance team. Gloria believes that accessibility should be a universal design.

V.G. VINOD VYDISWARAN is an associate professor of learning health sciences in the Medical School and associate professor of information in the School of Information, University of Michigan. His research is on natural language processing (NLP) algorithms, tools, and resources for medical informatics. His current research focuses on developing computable phenotypes, extracting clinically relevant information from electronic health record text, and federated network-based approaches to better train deep neural network models over health data.

D'SENA' WARREN is from Virginia by way of Florida. She is a mother of two boys, ages 14 and 10, and has lived with migraine attacks since childhood. Only after sustaining a traumatic brain injury in a motor vehicle accident in 2010 did she become chronic. She suffers daily from migraines along with a host of other comorbidities that affect her daily living. D'Sena' works to advocate for persons of color in a space that tends to push them off. When she is not working or advocating, she enjoys trying new foods with her boys.